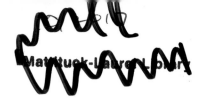
anatomy of exercise
FOR LONGEVITY

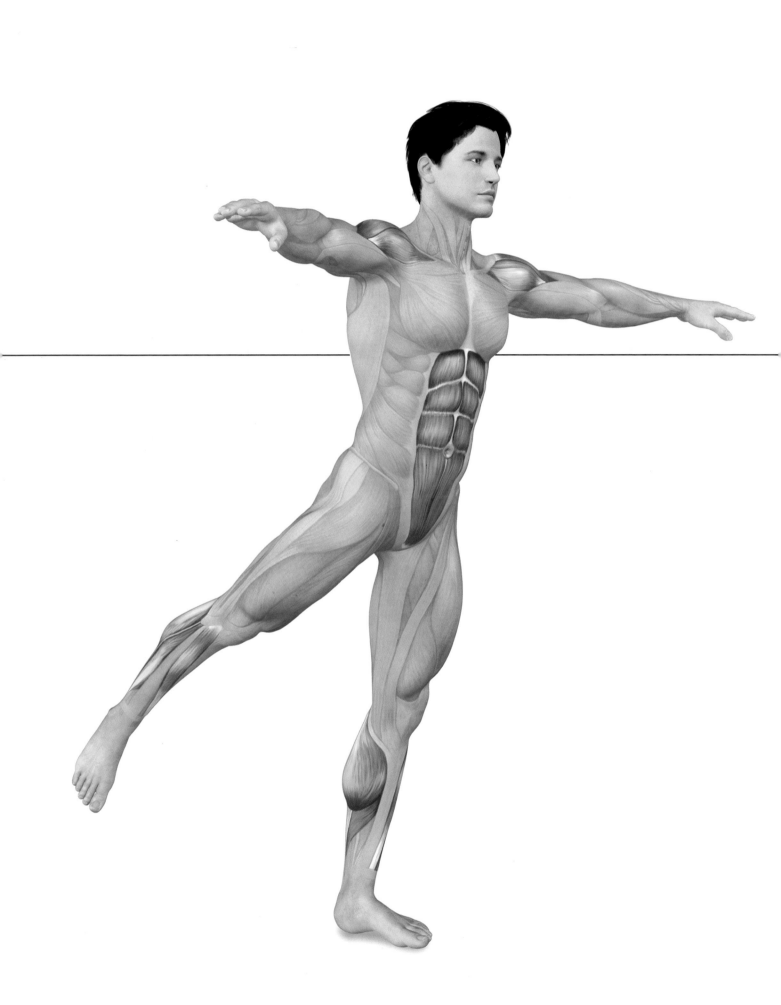

anatomy of exercise
FOR LONGEVITY

Hollis Lance Liebman

FIREFLY BOOKS

General Disclaimer

The contents of this book are intended to provide useful information to the general public. All materials, including texts, graphics, and images, are for informational purposes only and are not a substitute for medical diagnosis, advice, or treatment for specific medical conditions. All readers should seek expert medical care and consult their own physicians before commencing any exercise program or for any general or specific health issues. The author and publishers do not recommend or endorse specific treatments, procedures, advice, or other information found in this book and specifically disclaim all responsibility for any and all liability, loss, or risk, personal or otherwise, which is incurred as a consequence, directly or indirectly, of the use or application of any of the material in this publication.

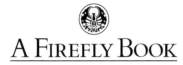

A FIREFLY BOOK

Published by Firefly Books Ltd. 2015

Copyright © 2015 Moseley Road Inc.

All rights reserved. No part of this publication may be reproduced, stored in a retrieval system, or transmitted in any form or by any means, electronic, mechanical, photocopying, recording or otherwise, without the prior written permission of the Publisher.

First printing

Publisher Cataloging-in-Publication Data (U.S.)

A CIP record for this title is available from the Library of Congress

Library and Archives Canada Cataloguing in Publication

A CIP record for this title is available from Library and Archives Canada

Published in the United States by
Firefly Books (U.S.) Inc.
P.O. Box 1338, Ellicott Station
Buffalo, New York 14205

Published in Canada by
Firefly Books Ltd.
50 Staples Avenue, Unit 1
Richmond Hill, Ontario L4B 0A7

Printed in Canada

Conceived, designed and produced by
Moseley Road Inc.
President: **Sean Moore**; General Manager: **Karen Prince**; Project Editor/
Designer: **Lisa Purcell Editorial & Design**; Production Designers: **Adam Moore**;
Photographer: **Jonathan Conklin Photography, Inc.**; Models: **BJ Gruber**,
David MacManamon, **Lou Matthews** and **Elaine Altholz**

CONTENTS

CONTENTS

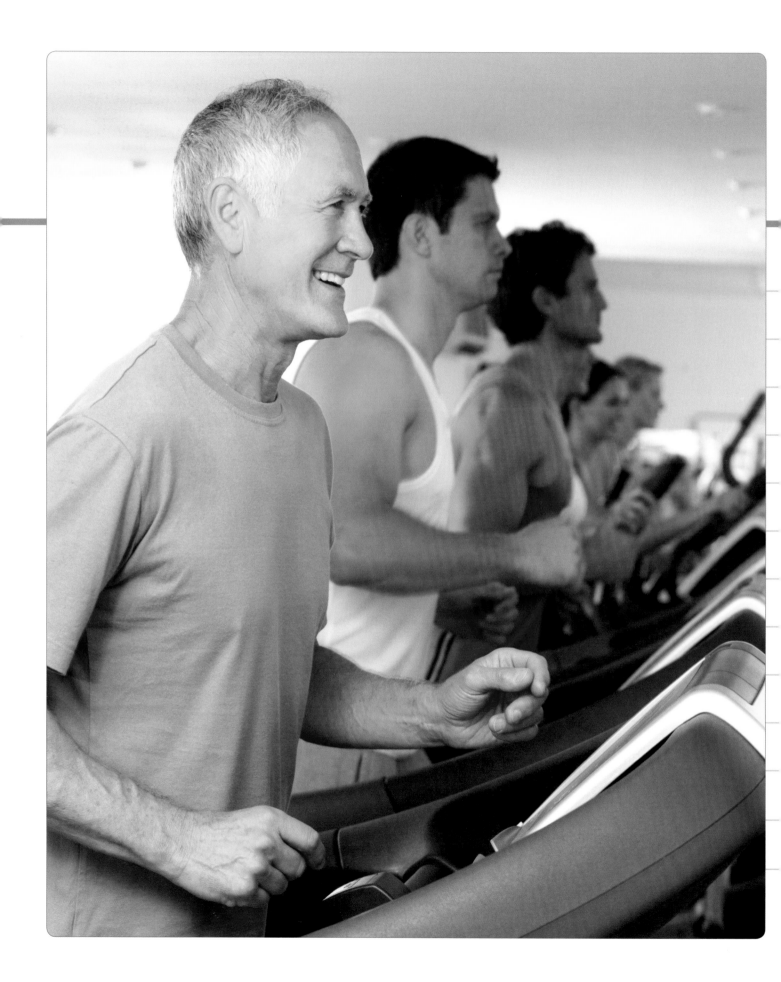

INTRODUCTION:
IN IT FOR
THE LONG HAUL

Longevity, defined as "a long duration of individual life," is something we all strive for—and we want not just a long life, but also a healthy one.

We want to be in it for the long haul.

Today we are seeing people living longer and, quite simply, living better. Advances in medicine have certainly improved our chances of making it to the century mark, but so too have advances in fitness and how we think about aging. No longer content to sit out our "declining" years, seniors are now jumping into the action. Now, more than ever before, parents and grandparents fill gyms and fitness centers, working out alongside their kids and grandkids. No longer does the sight of over-50s bench-lifting weights or bending into a complex yoga pose produce double-takes. Instead younger gym-goers are asking their elders how they too can look and feel as good.

IN IT FOR THE LONG HAUL

Fit older folks have learned that there comes a day when aesthetics (how the body looks), takes a back seat to functionality (how the body performs). When the question "How much can I bench?" is completely unimportant and replaced with "How do I feel?" As surely as we are seeing well-being and performance decline less—and sometimes even improve with a proper health and fitness regimen—living for the long haul with a high quality of life is rapidly becoming the norm.

Be it an injury, a stern warning from the doctor, a true glimpse into the mirror or any other such reason, there eventually does, however, come a point at which we simply can no longer do what we once did. We all eventually face the aging process. But what can keep this imminent process exciting rather than upsetting is the new goals that we can forge, along with a new way to achieve them. No longer have we accepted that aging equals permanent limitations or decline. What we have accepted is that working out, in addition to eating healthy, is truly the fountain of youth and will most certainly put the brakes on the aging process.

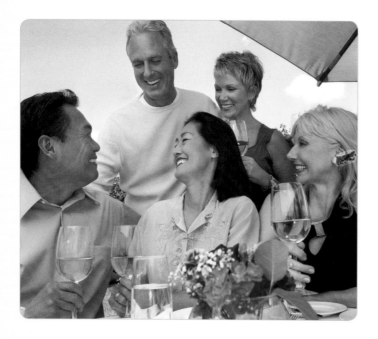

No matter what your age, it's never too late—nor too early—to begin longevity training. *Anatomy of Exercise for Longevity* isn't about honing a finely tuned athlete for a single event or peak performance—it's about improving your long-term well-being, whether you are 20 or 80. Longevity training can best be defined as the means of working toward an improved or maintained quality of physical life through a well-balanced program of fitness and nutrition. Longevity training will go beyond traditional weight training and include an equal measure of other longevity-boosting modalities, including strength training, postural/core exercises, mobility exercises, yoga exercises, cardio exercises, balance exercises and flexibility stretches. In other words, we are striving less toward forging big arms and more toward maintaining healthy hearts, good posture and flowing movement. The absolute takeaway is balance. The goal is to create a well-rounded individual who is not limited to merely being able to perform in the gym, but who also feels energetic and able-bodied out and about in daily life.

Imagine experiencing very little slowing down. Imagine living in less pain. And yes, imagine looking terrific at any age in your tank top, swimsuit and even in just your birthday suit. Imagine no longer, for this book is your key to becoming that person.

AGING

The term aging often brings with it a negative connotation. Too many of us tend to think of aging as a disease that comes with complications and limitations. But the truth is, genetics and, more important, lifestyle are major contributors to breaking through these preconceived limitations and living your second half to its fullest.

The out-dated stereotypical image of an older person severely limited and largely dependent on care is a thing of past. Three major action items—working out, good nutrition and recuperation—are essential to slowing down the effects of aging. These three things are well within your power, and although they will not permanently thwart the culprit that is aging, they will allow you to live your life to its fullest. Herein truly lives the fountain of youth. So why not take full advantage of it?

It is a fact that physical activity enhances life expectancy, and life expectancy is in fact what the true meaning of aging is. Take, for example, what happens when we meet a centenarian. "What's your secret?" is probably one of the first questions you ask a person who lives to be 100. And the answer is generally along the lines of living a stress-free life, keeping as active as possible, and avoiding a diet laden with processed foods and eating mostly natural foods.

So just what exactly is happening to your body during aging? What starts with a gray hair or a slight addition of fat around the midsection slowly continues on to bone and muscle loss, changes in posture, and cumulative aches and pains. Osteoporosis tends to affect women more than men, and this results in the loss of bone mass. In addition, the skin tends to lose its elasticity, bruising more easily and taking longer to heal. Aging also decreases the effectiveness of your body's immunity system—it slows down and you tend to take longer to heal.

Aging is the cumulative and ongoing process of physical and psychological change. Although physically you may slow down, mentally your brain and capacity for learning can keep growing. No matter what your chronological age, as long as certain diseases tend not to run genetically in your ancestry, you can begin the process of "successful aging" by remaining active and mentally inquisitive. Indeed, although we all must age, the "how" is largely up to us.

ANTI-AGING

Anti-aging is, of course, an oxymoron—we grow in age every second of every day, and aging is inevitable. But unlike a new car that depreciates the moment it is driven off the lot, the human body can improve long into its lifespan. Specialists now know that by introducing regular exercise, good nutrition and even regulating or reducing cortisol, the stress hormone, people are living a better quality of life, starting almost immediately. In truth, your second half of life can be your better half.

Research has shown that people who develop healthy habits improve their chances of living a long and active life. Regular exercise is a key, along with a clean nutritional intake composed of unrefined carbohydrates, good-quality fats (such as those found in salmon and avocados), lean protein (such as chicken and turkey breast), and vitamin, herb and antioxidant supplementation (such as calcium and vitamin D). Furthermore, controlling the release of insulin through diet can prevent or minimize your chances of such diseases as type 2 diabetes and can often even curtail or eliminate the use of prescription drugs. Exercise and nutrition are proactive measures directed toward fortifying your body, and they help you forestalling reactive measures such as relying on medications. You increase your chances of avoiding obesity and maintaining good health.

IN IT FOR THE LONG HAUL

THE ROLE OF SLEEP

These days, so many of us are sleep deprived. Sleep just seems to take a back seat to life and its many other priorities. Yet, lack of ample sleep effects not just alertness, but also your body's healing process as a whole. Lack of sleep, quality of sleep or simply enough sleep can result in changes in hormones and glucose tolerance, and the ongoing effects of sleep deprivation can even result in early stages of type 2 diabetes. The final stage of sleep—REM sleep, or deep sleep—is a natural anti-aging process that rejuvenates and restores your body from the effects of the daily grind and is the final stage of sleep. If you strive each night to get quality REM sleep, then you are well onto your way in slowing down and even reversing the aging process.

STRESS REDUCTION AND LONGEVITY

We all know that stress is a negative factor, not only in terms of overall longevity but also in our day-to-day existence. Stress effects your body's ability to relax and amply repair and rejuvenate itself. During times of stress our bodies can release the hormone cortisol, which has been labeled "the stress hormone." The role of cortisol is to activate anti-stress and anti-inflammatory pathways, and it can have positive benefits such as lower pain sensitivity, heightened memory and quick bursts of energy for urgent bodily functioning and survival. Prolonged or chronic stress, however, can result in cortisol remaining in the bloodstream for too long, which can cause a decrease in muscle mass and bone density, high blood pressure,

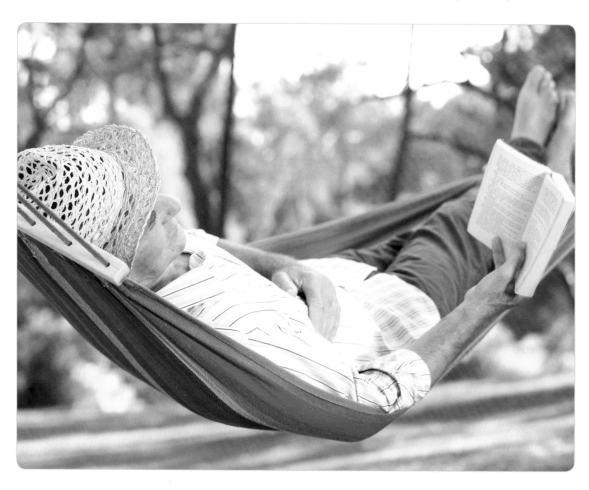

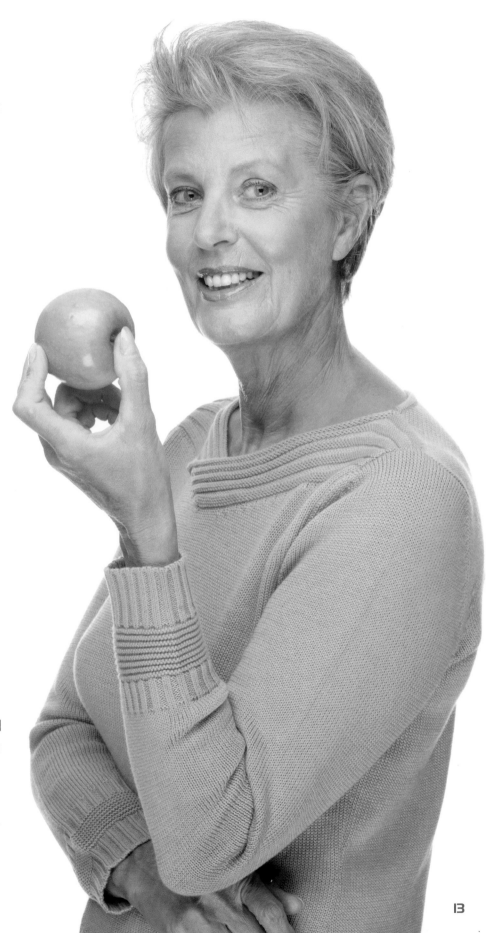

lowered immunity and increased body fat—all leading to further health problems.

Stress and cortisol levels can be kept in check and under control by maintaining a regular lifestyle that includes exercise and healthful nutrition, as well as keeping the mind healthy. Learning stress-management techniques and not turning to high-glycemic carbohydrates during times of great stress will add both years and quality to your life—and it goes down far better than any donut or bread ever could.

NUTRITION

As history and science has shown us, what we consume has a profound and direct effect on not only how we look, but on how we feel. The old adage "You are what you eat" is absolutely true. Eating foods that are largely unprocessed will not only help to keep you lean, but will also supply the fuel you need to lead an active and productive life. Sticking to mainly the outer perimeters of the supermarket, with its raw and fresher foods, will help to ensure better choices.

Avoiding the processed foods that occupy the vast majority of the center aisles of your supermarket will allow your body to actually process fuel more efficiently due to the naturally occurring fiber content contained in fresh fruits and vegetables. Processed foods are largely devoid of fiber and are often infused with sugar, which causes your body to release insulin, the fat storage hormone. Insulin is rapidly released from the pancreas in an effort to defensively and immediately deal with the intake of sugar, which is shuttled into fat cells, resulting in a heavier, less healthy person. As age goes up, risks for diseases such as type 2 diabetes can increase for those not paying attention to what's on their plate or their weekly schedule of activities.

Consuming a nutritional intake of slow-burning, long-term-energy-producing

IN IT FOR THE LONG HAUL

carbohydrates, such as beans and other legumes, brown rice, quinoa, oatmeal and yams will help to ensure optimal energy levels and a steady, nonspiking release of sugar.

What many forget in regard to nutrition is that carbs, be they in the form of fruits, vegetables, or salads, are broken down and used in the body primarily as energy. And the same goes for the calorie-dense macronutrient fat. Both contain, at best, trace amounts of protein.

Good sources of fats are those found in raw nuts, avocados, olives and salmon. Consumed daily and in moderation, they will help to keep you satiated as they strengthen and enhance your skin, hair, heart and joints.

It is amino acids, the building blocks of muscle (or protein) that must also be consumed but are often neglected, and they are truly what we are made of. You must consume muscle to build and even maintain muscle. Eggs, chicken, turkey, fish and lean cuts of beef are excellent sources of protein and will help to keep you strong and even firm well into your upper ages.

Science and application has shown that four to five small, nonprocessed meals per day are far more effective for energy maintenance well into your later years. The old guide for three square meals a day that are heavily reliant on processed carbohydrates such as breads, cereals and pastas is an ineffective and outdated system.

Additionally, in order to keep insulin levels in check, always consume a low-fat protein source with your low-glycemic carbohydrates in order to keep the effect on your blood sugar minimal and keep body fat at bay.

Along with the exercise program outlined in this book, there are a number of actions you can take in order to make your nutritional lifestyle work for you. Rather than trying to keep to an onerous diet that you will ultimately break, begin a plan of smart eating that you can stick to for the long haul. Here a few tips:

- Prepare healthy meals the night or even days before and store or pack them. This simple measure will help to ensure that you do not skip meals or become a slave to availability. If you have something prepared in advance or packed with you on the road, you won't be tempted to make poor choices when in a bind. You can also carry with you meal replacement shakes.
- Never food shop or head out to parties when you are hungry: a hungry person makes bad nutritional choices. Before setting out for the supermarket or a social event, eat a light and healthy meal. You will be less tempted by low-value snacks.

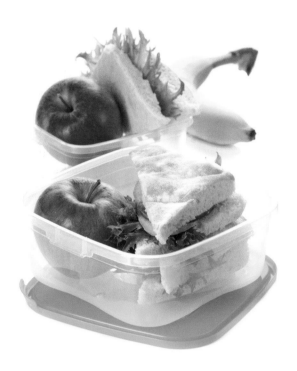

HYDRATION

Staying hydrated is essential to your well-being and survival. We know that our bodies are largely composed of water, and our organs, tissues and cells must have water in order to function. Most of us have been told that we should be consuming at least eight glasses of water per day. If you are an active person, simply drinking whenever you feel thirsty will replace the fluids lost during sweating, exercise and even breathing. Water is the best source for staying hydrated because it is pure, but there are other options.

You can consume teas, vegetable and fruit juices, and even milk—sparingly, provided you're not lactose intolerant. It is important to consider calorie content and, in particular, sugar content, which is often high in fruit juices especially. Limit your intake of sports drinks because they not only often contain a lot of sugar, but they also sometimes contain stimulants that are might be harmful to those with an intolerance or sensitivity.

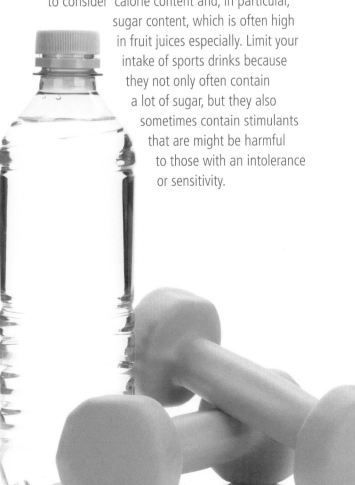

- Rid your home of processed foods. This will make it harder for you to give in to sudden and strong temptation. You can simply toss out foods that aren't going to support you and your healthy lifestyle or donate them. Stock your pantry and refrigerator with a variety of healthy and tasty foods that will offer a variety of choices, be palatably sound, and, above all, support your longevity lifestyle.

- Learn to make healthy choice selections when dining out. Socializing is a part of life but just because you are out to dinner, does not mean you should completely give in to temptation or follow the masses with eating foods that don't support your goals. Just about any restaurant or cuisine offers a healthier alternative on their menu, and chances are high that if a good choice doesn't appear on the menu, the establishment can generally accommodate a healthy and clean off-the-menu request.

IN IT FOR THE LONG HAUL

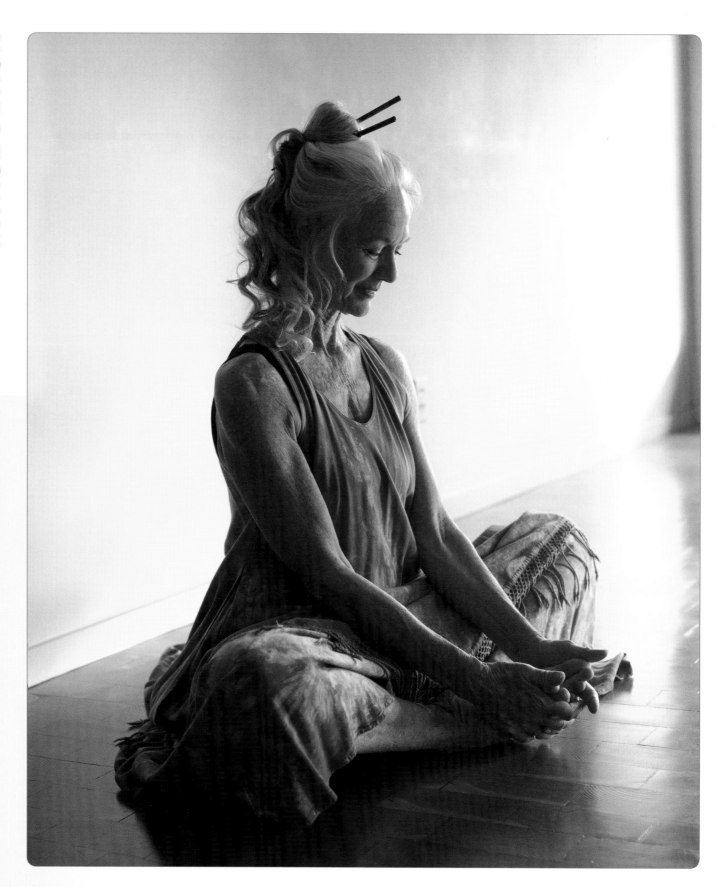

THE SEVEN MODALITIES OF LONGEVITY TRAINING

The previously mentioned seven exercise modalities—strength training, postural/core exercises, mobility exercises, yoga exercises, cardio exercises, balance exercises and flexibility stretches—form your well-rounded and optimal fitness routine. Again, a program that offers optimal health, functionality and longevity requires more than a routine spin on the old stationary bike or even a light jog or brisk-paced treadmill session.

These seven modalities, although all are an integral part of your longevity program, are placed in order of importance and sequencing in your workout.

1. Strength Training

In addition to building muscle and elevating your metabolism (the more muscle mass the more calories one burns at rest), there are too many benefits to weight training to ignore. For those with a heart condition or arthritis, strength training can be a huge plus by strengthening bones, reducing pain and improving heart function. It may even reverse both bone and muscle loss. Strength training also helps to sculpt or shape your body in ways that cardiovascular exercise cannot, in addition to reducing your risk of falling as you get older. Resistance training can also lift your mood and has been proven effective against some forms of depression.

2. Postural/Core Exercises

The core, composed of multiple muscle groups, including your pelvic and hip muscles, lower-back muscles and abdominal muscles, provides support for all body movement. Any fitness program must include a core focus because strenghtening these muscles will result in better posture, stability, alignment and more.

3. Mobility Exercises

Reading like a who's who list of benefits, the advantages of mobility training has earned this modality its rightful place in the longevity repertoire. Movement practice helps move a joint through a full range of motion (ROM) and active flexibility, helps in removing toxins and reduces joint pain and inflammation. It can prolong or add years of life to strong working joints. Devoting just minutes a day to mobility exercises can result in greater health and longevity. Differing from stretching in that it targets all movement-restricting elements as opposed to just lengthening short and tight muscles, mobility training is injury prevention and insurance that the proper joints are firing during exercise performance.

4. Yoga Exercises

Long-term yoga practitioners have reported elevated moods and mental clarity (less anxiety), as well as muscular and strength improvements. This modality offers many benefits, including but not limited to improved balance, posture, coordination, flexibility and core strength. In other words, yoga is simply too effective to pass up. It is superb for stretching tight and restricted muscles, as well as improving actual muscle tone and even in reducing blood pressure. It can be performed just about anywhere with no special equipment, and you can adapt it to any age, body type and skill level.

IN IT FOR THE LONG HAUL

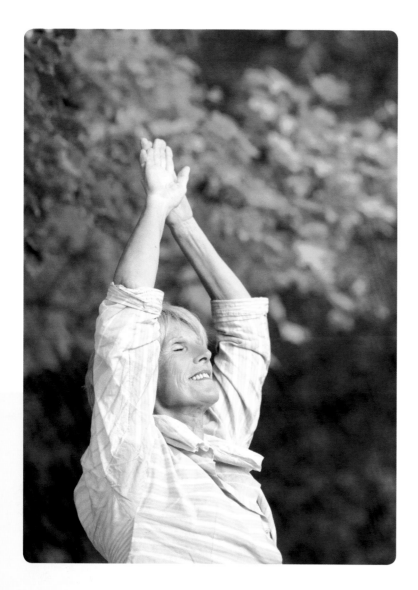

paralyzing effects of depression. Endurance activities are the perfect complement to anaerobic activities, such as strength training, offering you a wide and complete array of health benefits. Cardiovascular exercise in its purest sense is best performed following resistance training. Too often, performing all-out high-intensity cardio prior to other forms of exercise leaves you too tired to complete your fitness routine. And in some cases, cardio leaves you ravenous and subject to bad food choices.

6. Balance Exercises

All functional movements require proper balance. Balance training helps to both develop and maintain your ability to correctly hold your body's position, which helps to prevent accidental falls. This modality improves dynamic joint stabilization, which keeps joints aligned during movement. It also strengthens your core and improves your body's stability, coordination and strength. Balance exercises can be performed nearly anywhere and at any time and can be modified to suit any needs.

7. Flexibility Stretches

As youths, we are taught in gym class to stretch prior to activity. We learn as adults to get up every once in a while and shake it out, especially if we have a largely sedentary vocation. And animals instinctively do it prior to movement and upon waking up. Aside from increasing flexibility and range of motion, regular stretching improves your circulation and cardiovascular health and even helps to alleviate some pain. Despite what we learned in gym class, in practice it is best to avoid stretching before exercise because your muscles are not yet warm and pliable. You should instead stretch both during and after exercise. Overstretching prior to being warmed up can be counterproductive and even result in injury.

5. Cardio Exercises

The term *cardiovascular*, or simply *cardio*, refers to a continuous activity involving the heart and the presence of oxygen. In addition to helping to keep the heart (also a muscle) strong and promoting blood circulation, cardiovascular exercise helps to elevate the metabolism, that is the rate at which calories are burned. It will also help you build endurance for athletic pursuits and your daily tasks.

The continual implementation of cardio training also promotes the release of "feel-good" hormones that promote a sense of well-being and help to thwart the sometimes

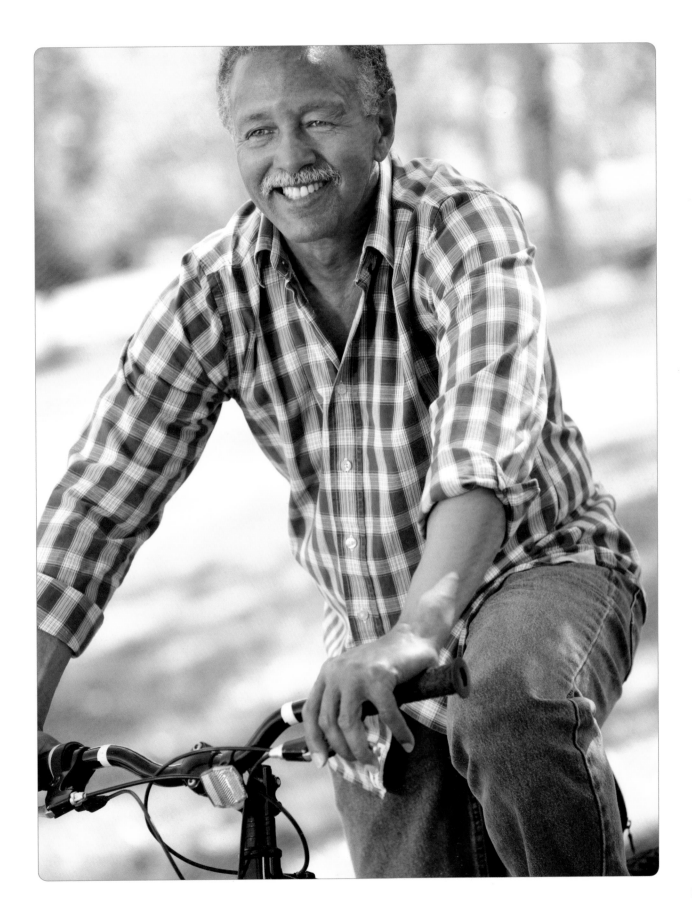

IN IT FOR THE LONG HAUL

PUTTING IT ALL TOGETHER

Just as there exists a direct correlation between the fuel put into a car and how it ultimately performs, the same can be said of the human body. If you live a life devoid of exercise or movement and consume largely processed foods, then your body will at best respond by prematurely aging. But if you live your life with regular exercise and support that movement with sound nutrition, then you are going to very gradually feel the aging process. You will be able to do things—and do them well into your later years. It's that simple.

One of the great benefits about performing the longevity program is its portability and bare-bones approach. It will take just minutes a day to get the most from it, and you can perform the entire protocol at your home or in your office and with very little specialized gear. There's no need to join your local gym (although you most certainly can if the urge strikes you), because the equipment needed is indeed minimal. A Swiss ball, dumbbells or hand weights and resistance

How to Use This Book
In the step-by-step chapters of this book, you'll find photos with instructions demonstrating how to execute each exercise and some tips on what to do to perform it correctly—and what to avoid. Some exercises have accompanying variations, shown in the modification box. Alongside each exercise is a quick-read panel that lists the exercise's major target, level of difficulty, and benefits. Also included is a list of precautions: if you have one of the issues listed, it is best to avoid that exercise. Each exercise also features illustrations showing key muscles. As you work out, visualize the muscles that you are engaging—it will help you maintain optimal form.

bands will get you well on your way toward living a better quality of life.

Along with the detailed descriptions contained after each exercise about correct performance and usage, and the differing types of workouts to follow later in the book, you will also need to support your protocol with some form of direct cardiovascular exercise. This will support your heart and fat-burning efforts as well as help you to more efficiently perform the anaerobic portion of your exercise routine.

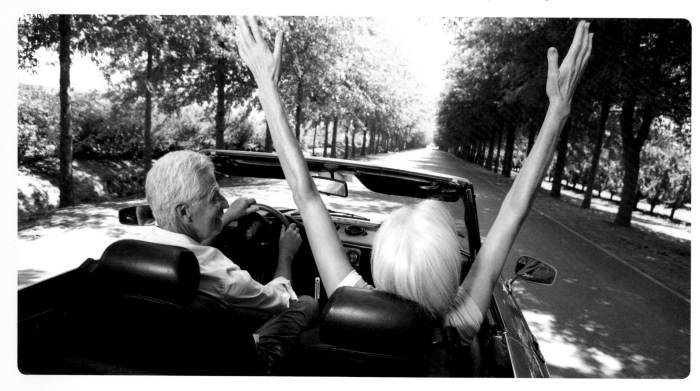

BEST FOR

Many of the featured exercises incorporate equipment—all reasonably small tools that add variety and challenge to your workout.

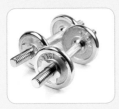

Dumbbells and hand weights. Strength-training exercises often call for dumbbells or other weights. You can start with very light, 2 pound (.9 kg) hand weights (or even lighter substitutes, such as unopened food cans or water bottles), and then work your way up to heavier ones. Both hand weights and dumbbells add resistance, increasing the benefits of many exercises. You can use either one for any exercise that calls for a weight. If you decide to invest in a set of dumbbells, look for an adjustable model that allows you to easily vary the weight levels. Be sure it comes with a solid-locking mechanism that makes adding and subtracting weight disks fast and easy.

Swiss ball. Also known as an exercise ball, fitness ball, body ball, or balance ball, this heavy-duty inflatable ball is available in a variety of sizes, with diameters ranging from 18 to 30 inches (45–76 cm). Be sure to find the best size for your height and weight. A Swiss ball is an excellent fitness aid that really works your core. Because it is unstable, you must constantly adjust your balance while performing a movement, which helps you improve your overall sense of balance and your flexibility.

Resistance bands. Also known as "fitness band," "Thera-Band," "Dyna-Band," "stretching band," and "exercise band," this simple tool adds resistance to an exercise. You will see two types of resistance bands, one with handles and one without; both are amazing pieces of fitness equipment, which effectively tone and strengthen your entire body. Bands act in a similar way to hand weights, but unlike weights, which rely on gravity to determine the resistance, bands use constant tension—supplied by your muscles—to add resistance to your movements and improve your overall coordination.

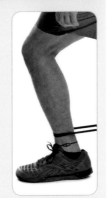

Studies have shown that performing continuous cardiovascular exercise for a minimum of three times a week for 20 minutes consecutively produces a positive effect on metabolism. Be it hiking, jogging on a treadmill, stationary cycling and on and on ad infinitum, cardio involves your heart and will help to add years of quality to your life.

The workout modalities to follow are full-body in nature, as opposed to a traditional bodybuilding or strength-training protocol in which one or two specific muscles are worked for that particular day in an effort to create maximum size and strength. The nontraditional full-body format provides you with a stronger, firmer and more functional body overall.

Chances are you won't be asked to flex your arm or show off your chest development (although you may), but just ask yourself how amazing it will feel to lift boxes around the house effortlessly and pain-free. Or to actually get a full night's sleep and awake rejuvenated and energetic instead of exhausted and hurting.

The longevity program is well-rounded and geared toward incremental improvements over time. It is not just about maintenance—it is a non-impactful program that will preserve your joints and mobility while strengthening and freeing them.

LIFE BALANCE

Longevity truly starts with the mind. If you picture yourself aging with a host of ailments and a drawer full of medications to manage them, then that could be your future. But if you aspire to live a life that is active and fulfilling, aspire to play ball with your children and their children, aspire to be mobile until the end, then program your mind to make it a reality.

If you're reading this book, then you believe that the only limitations are self-imposed and that your quality of life is far less contingent on what others deem limiting, and much more about you, your abilities and how far you are willing to go. How far is that? Dare to venture to your exponential limits and find out.

FULL-BODY ANATOMY

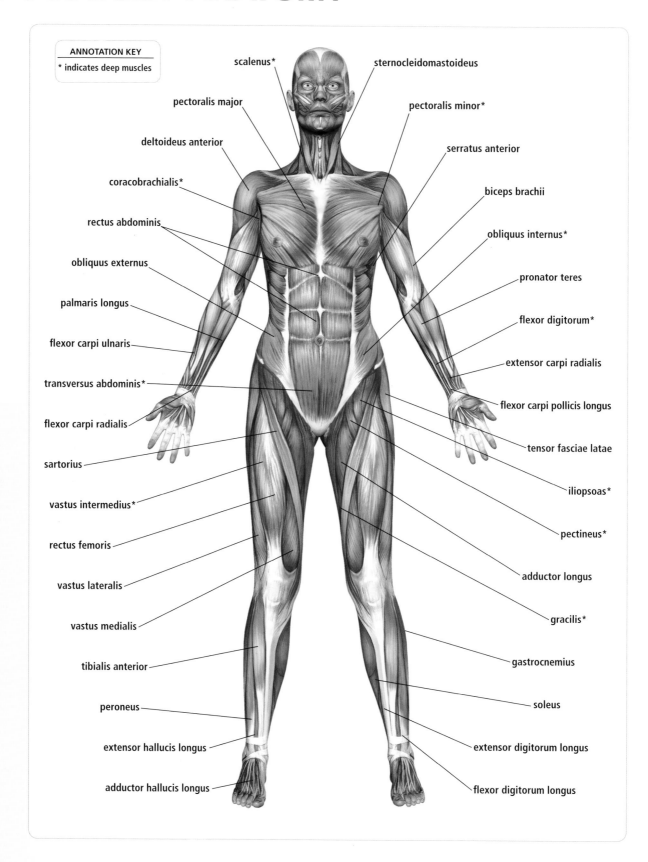

ANNOTATION KEY
* indicates deep muscles

scalenus*

sternocleidomastoideus

pectoralis major

pectoralis minor*

deltoideus anterior

serratus anterior

coracobrachialis*

biceps brachii

rectus abdominis

obliquus internus*

obliquus externus

pronator teres

palmaris longus

flexor digitorum*

flexor carpi ulnaris

extensor carpi radialis

transversus abdominis*

flexor carpi pollicis longus

flexor carpi radialis

tensor fasciae latae

sartorius

iliopsoas*

vastus intermedius*

pectineus*

rectus femoris

adductor longus

vastus lateralis

gracilis*

vastus medialis

gastrocnemius

tibialis anterior

soleus

peroneus

extensor hallucis longus

extensor digitorum longus

adductor hallucis longus

flexor digitorum longus

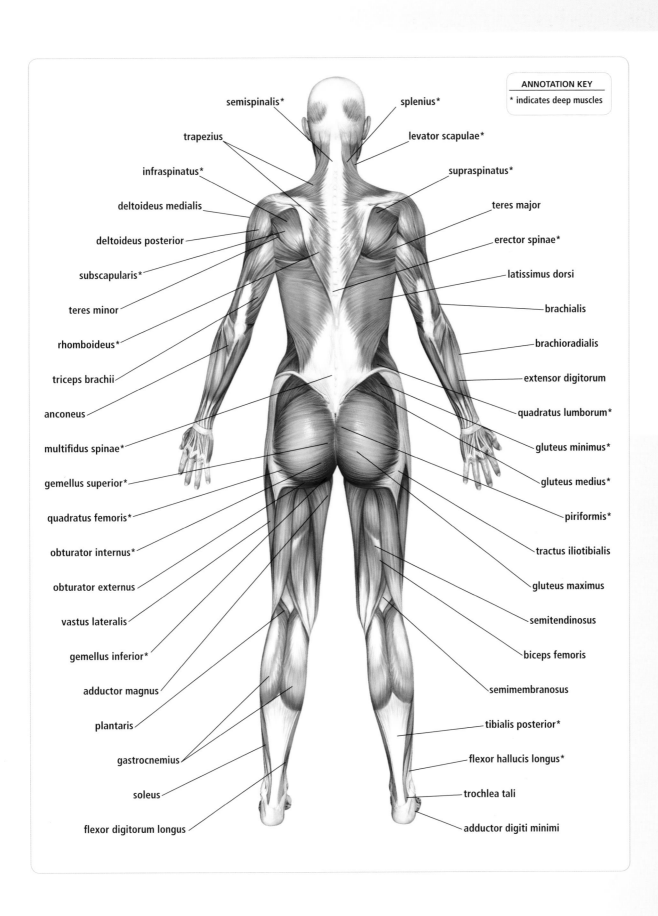

ANNOTATION KEY
* indicates deep muscles

semispinalis*

splenius*

trapezius

levator scapulae*

infraspinatus*

suddenly supraspinatus*

deltoideus medialis

teres major

deltoideus posterior

erector spinae*

subscapularis*

latissimus dorsi

teres minor

brachialis

rhomboideus*

brachioradialis

triceps brachii

extensor digitorum

anconeus

quadratus lumborum*

multifidus spinae*

gluteus minimus*

gemellus superior*

gluteus medius*

quadratus femoris*

piriformis*

obturator internus*

tractus iliotibialis

obturator externus

gluteus maximus

vastus lateralis

semitendinosus

gemellus inferior*

biceps femoris

adductor magnus

semimembranosus

plantaris

tibialis posterior*

gastrocnemius

flexor hallucis longus*

soleus

trochlea tali

flexor digitorum longus

adductor digiti minimi

23

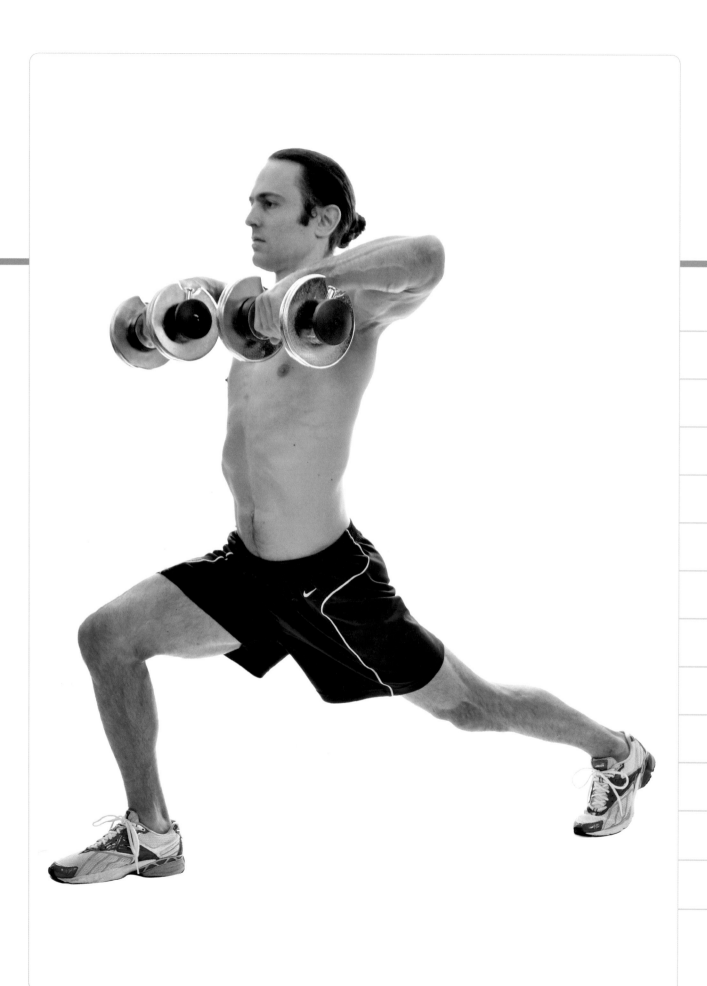

STRENGTH TRAINING

Strength training, also known as resistance training, is a major component

of a longevity workout. Geared to building and toning muscles, this part of

your workout has multiple benefits. Building stronger muscles improves their

functionality, making physical tasks, such as lifting and carrying, far easier—no

matter what your age. Strength training will also help prevent muscle strain

and pain—for example, a stronger back can tolerate far more stress, which

reduces the chance of injury. It has also been shown to help fortify against the

bone loss and weakening of osteoporosis.

The following exercises target various important muscle groups, enhancing

their size, strength and functionality. In some cases, exercises have been

combined to get the absolute most in terms of efficiency and effectiveness

from your longevity training.

SWISS BALL SQUAT WITH DUMBBELL CURL

❶ Place a Swiss ball against a wall and stand with your back to it so that your middle to lower back is pinning the Swiss ball to the wall. Your feet should be about hip-width apart and slightly forward of your hips. Grasp a pair of dumbbells in each hand with your palms facing forward.

❷ Bend your knees and descend until your thighs are parallel to the floor while simultaneously bending your arms until your palms are nearly touching the front of your shoulders.

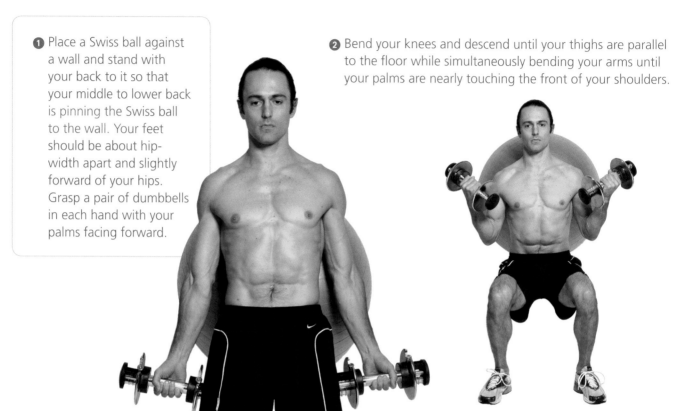

TARGETS
• Quadriceps
• Glutes
• Biceps

LEVEL
• Beginner

BENEFITS
• Strengthens thighs and upper arms

NOT ADVISABLE IF YOU HAVE . . .
• Knee issues

❸ Straighten your legs as you bring your arms down to return to the starting position.

❹ Reset and then repeat for 12 to 15 repetitions

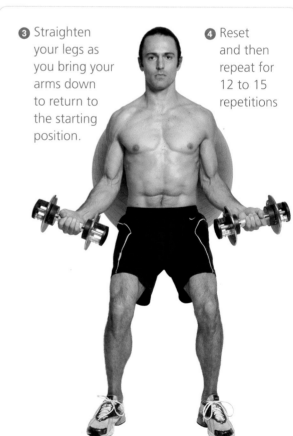

DO IT RIGHT
• Lower just until the tops of your thighs are parallel to the floor.
• Flex your biceps at the top of the movement.

AVOID
• Hyperextending your knees past your toes.

MODIFICATION
Easier: Use just your body weight.

BEST FOR
- rectus femoris
- vastus lateralis
- vastus intermedius
- vastus medialis
- gluteus maximus

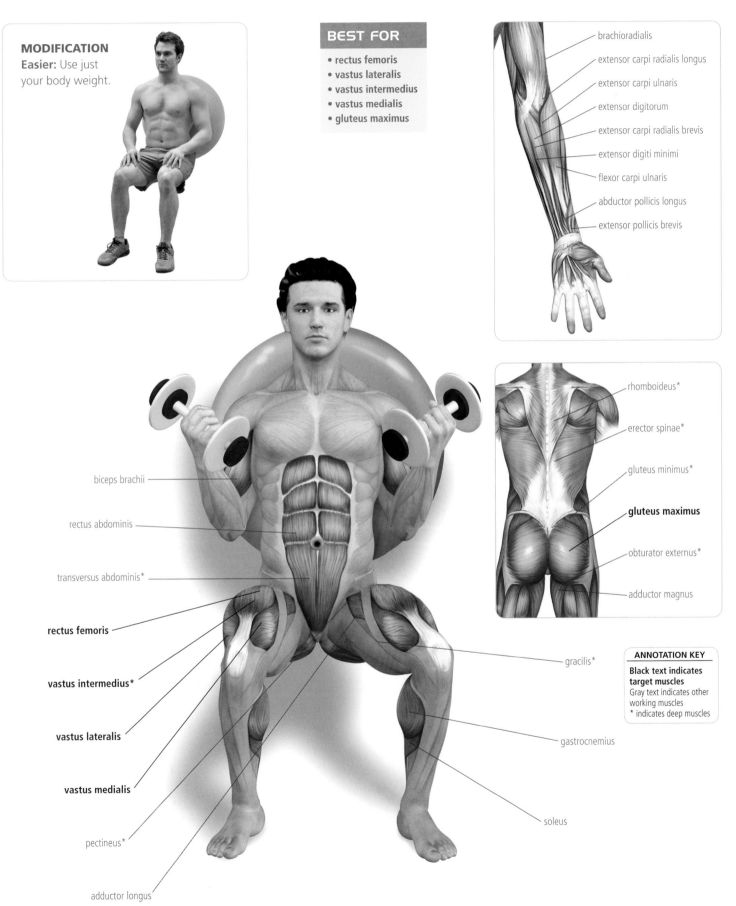

brachioradialis

extensor carpi radialis longus

extensor carpi ulnaris

extensor digitorum

extensor carpi radialis brevis

extensor digiti minimi

flexor carpi ulnaris

abductor pollicis longus

extensor pollicis brevis

biceps brachii

rectus abdominis

transversus abdominis*

rectus femoris

vastus intermedius*

vastus lateralis

vastus medialis

pectineus*

adductor longus

gracilis*

gastrocnemius

soleus

rhomboideus*

erector spinae*

gluteus minimus*

gluteus maximus

obturator externus*

adductor magnus

ANNOTATION KEY

Black text indicates target muscles
Gray text indicates other working muscles
* indicates deep muscles

LUNGE WITH DUMBBELL UPRIGHT ROW

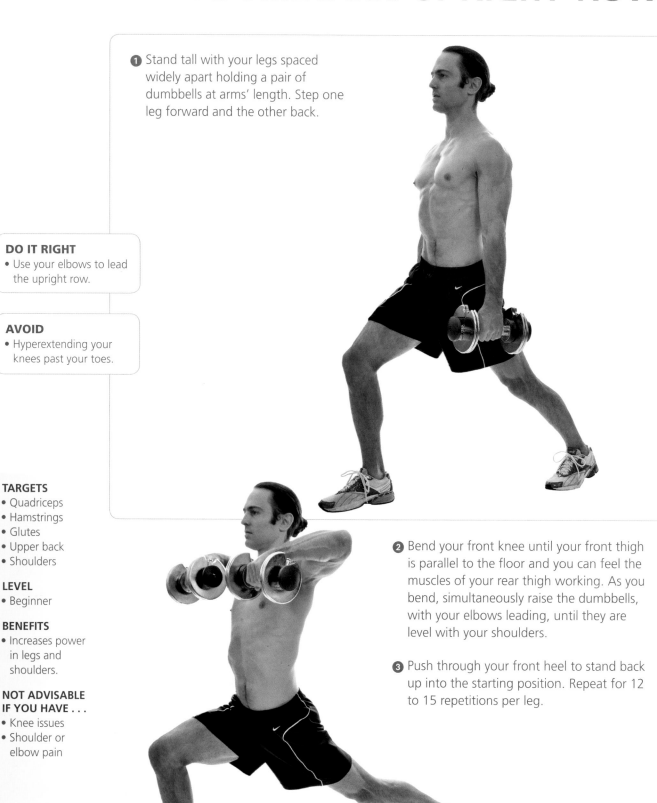

❶ Stand tall with your legs spaced widely apart holding a pair of dumbbells at arms' length. Step one leg forward and the other back.

DO IT RIGHT
• Use your elbows to lead the upright row.

AVOID
• Hyperextending your knees past your toes.

TARGETS
• Quadriceps
• Hamstrings
• Glutes
• Upper back
• Shoulders

LEVEL
• Beginner

BENEFITS
• Increases power in legs and shoulders.

NOT ADVISABLE IF YOU HAVE . . .
• Knee issues
• Shoulder or elbow pain

❷ Bend your front knee until your front thigh is parallel to the floor and you can feel the muscles of your rear thigh working. As you bend, simultaneously raise the dumbbells, with your elbows leading, until they are level with your shoulders.

❸ Push through your front heel to stand back up into the starting position. Repeat for 12 to 15 repetitions per leg.

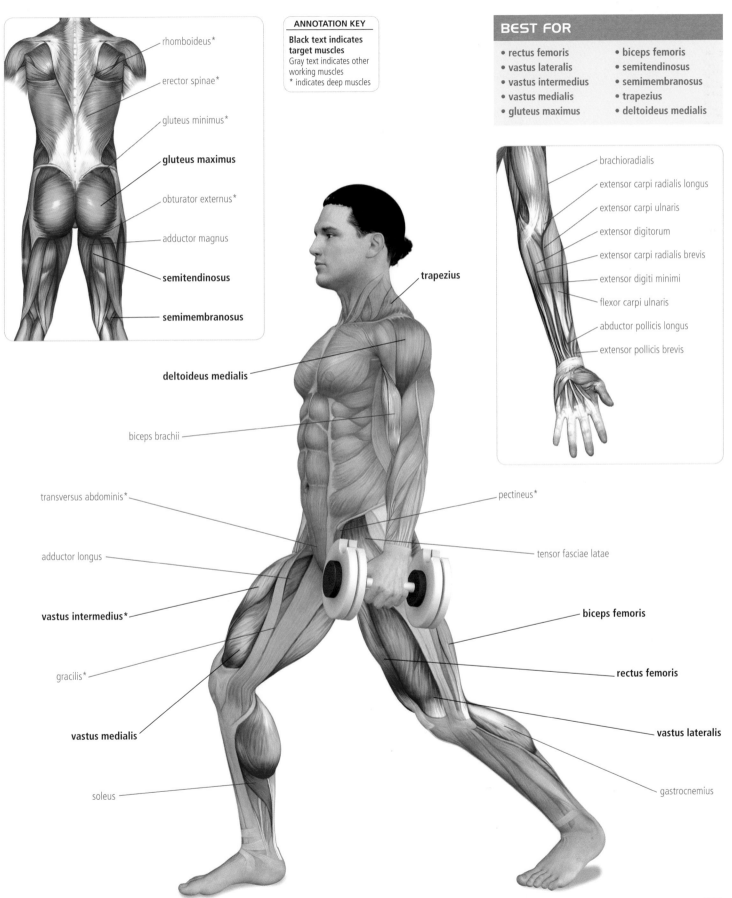

ANNOTATION KEY

Black text indicates
target muscles
Gray text indicates other
working muscles
* indicates deep muscles

BEST FOR

- rectus femoris
- vastus lateralis
- vastus intermedius
- vastus medialis
- gluteus maximus
- biceps femoris
- semitendinosus
- semimembranosus
- trapezius
- deltoideus medialis

rhomboideus*

erector spinae*

gluteus minimus*

gluteus maximus

obturator externus*

adductor magnus

semitendinosus

semimembranosus

trapezius

brachioradialis

extensor carpi radialis longus

extensor carpi ulnaris

extensor digitorum

extensor carpi radialis brevis

extensor digiti minimi

flexor carpi ulnaris

abductor pollicis longus

extensor pollicis brevis

deltoideus medialis

biceps brachii

transversus abdominis*

pectineus*

adductor longus

tensor fasciae latae

vastus intermedius*

biceps femoris

gracilis*

rectus femoris

vastus medialis

vastus lateralis

soleus

gastrocnemius

SWISS BALL INCLINE DUMBBELL PRESS

❶ Lie face-up on a Swiss ball, with your upper back, neck and head supported. Keep your torso elongated, and bend your knees at a right angle. Plant your feet on the floor a little wider than shoulder-distance apart. Grasp a hand weight or dumbbell in each hand, and bend your elbows so that the weights are in line with your shoulders.

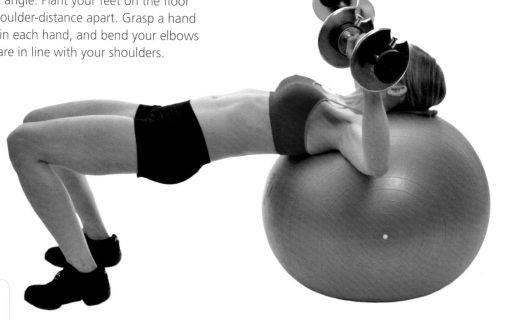

AVOID
• Bouncing the weight off your chest.
• Allowing your lower back to sag.

TARGETS
• Chest
• Core

LEVEL
• Intermediate

BENEFITS
• Strengthens pectoral muscles
• Strengthens and stabilizes core

NOT ADVISABLE IF YOU HAVE . . .
• Shoulder issues
• Lower-back issues

❷ Drop your rear slightly so that your torso takes on an "incline" position.

❸ Press your arms upward until they are straight.

❹ Bend your elbows as you lower the weights toward your shoulders back to the starting postion. Repeat, performing three sets of 15.

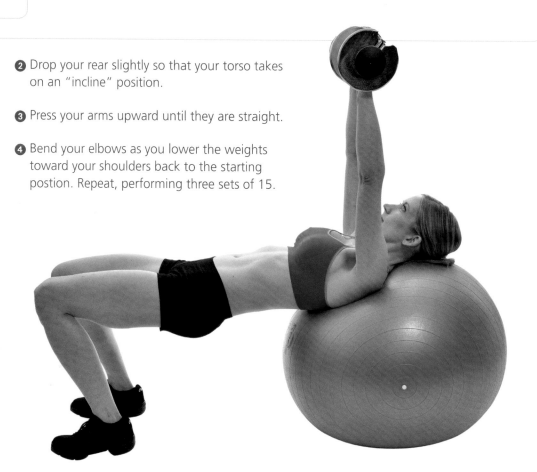

DO IT RIGHT
- Lower the weights with control.
- Keep your heels firmly pressed into the floor.
- Keep your wrists in line with your shoulders.

BEST FOR
- pectoralis major
- pectoralis minor

deltoideus medialis

deltoideus posterior

erector spinae*

ANNOTATION KEY
Black text indicates target muscles
Gray text indicates other working muscles
* indicates deep muscles

pectoralis minor*

pectoralis major

rectus abdominis

transversus abdominis*

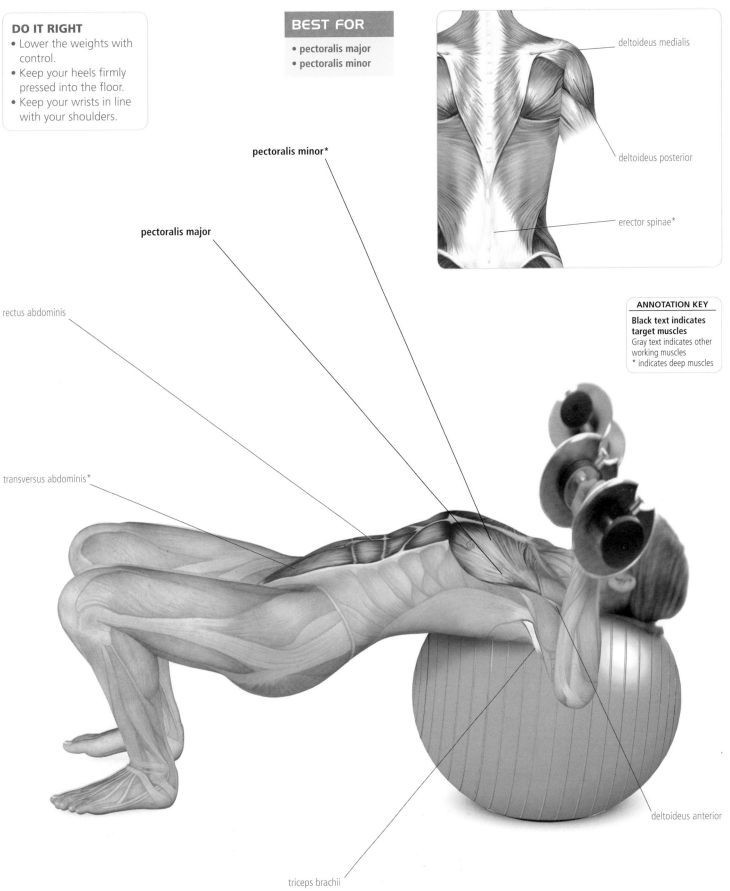

triceps brachii

deltoideus anterior

SWISS BALL DUMBBELL PULLOVER

❶ Lie face-up on a Swiss ball, with your upper back, neck and head supported. Your body should be extended with your torso long, knees bent at a right angle and feet planted on the floor a little wider than shoulder-distance apart. Grasp a hand weight or dumbbell in each hand, and extend your arms behind you, level with your shoulders so that your body from knees to fingertips forms a straight line.

AVOID
• Locking your arms when they are extended behind your head.
• Arching your back.
• Rushing through the exercise.

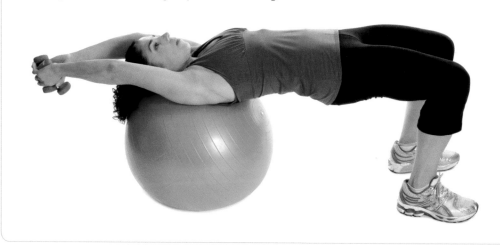

❷ Keeping the rest of your body stable and your arms as straight as possible, raise your arms upward so that they are perpendicular to your body.

❸ Return your arms to starting position. Repeat for 12 to 15 repetitions.

TARGETS
• Upper back
• Core

LEVEL
• Intermediate

BENEFITS
• Strengthens upper back
• Stabilizes core

NOT ADVISABLE IF YOU HAVE . . .
• Shoulder issues

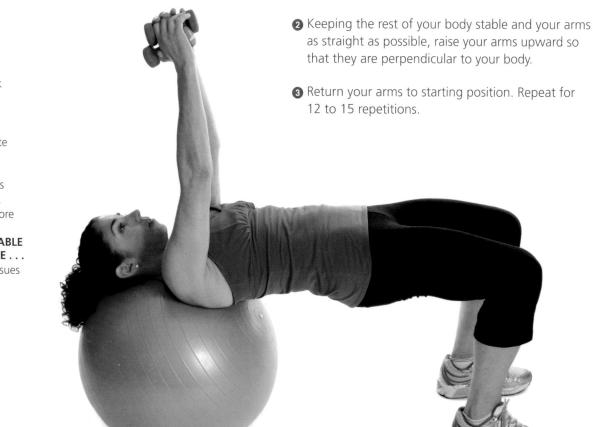

BEST FOR
• latissimus dorsi
• serratus anterior

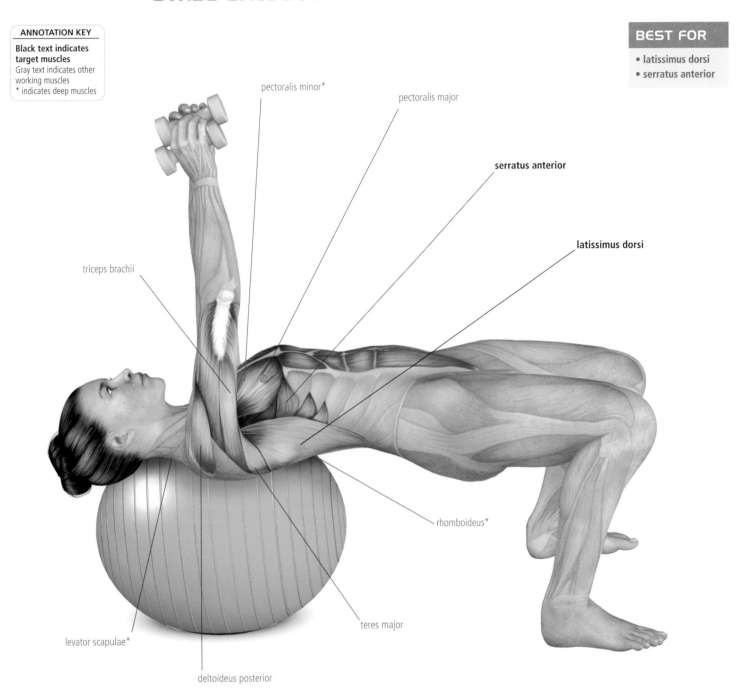

pectoralis minor*

pectoralis major

serratus anterior

latissimus dorsi

triceps brachii

rhomboideus*

teres major

levator scapulae*

deltoideus posterior

DO IT RIGHT
• Ease into the movement.
• Keep your arms directly above your shoulders when lifting the weights overhead.
• Keep your torso stable and feet planted throughout the exercise.
• Engage your abs.
• Keep your buttocks and pelvis lifted so that your upper legs, torso and neck form a straight line.
• Move your arms smoothly and with control.

MODIFICATION
Similar level of difficulty:
Grasp a single dumbbell with both hands.

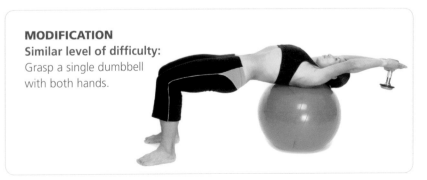

SEATED ALTERNATING DUMBBELL PRESS

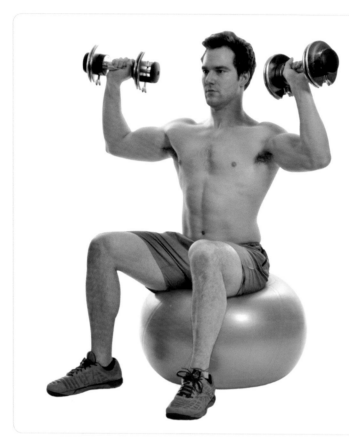

1 Sit on a Swiss ball in a well-balanced, neutral position, with your hips directly over the center of the ball, grasping a dumbbell in each hand. Hold one to each side of your shoulders with your elbows below your wrists.

TARGETS
• Shoulders

LEVEL
• Beginner

BENEFITS
• Strengthens shoulders and upper back

NOT ADVISABLE IF YOU HAVE . . .
• Shoulder issues
• Rotator cuff injury

2 Press one arm upward to full lockout, and then lower down the same pathway.

AVOID
• Lowering too far outside your shoulders.
• Tensing your neck.
• Wiggling or squirming in an effort to press the weights upward.

3 Repeat on the other arm, and then continue to alternate sides for a total of 12 to 15 repetitions per arm.

rhomboideus*

erector spinae*

ANNOTATION KEY

Black text indicates target muscles
Gray text indicates other working muscles
* indicates deep muscles

BEST FOR

• deltoideus anterior

deltoideus medialis

deltoideus anterior

rectus abdominis

trapezius

triceps brachii

DO IT RIGHT
• Keep your movements slow and controlled.
• Pause at the top of the movement, and then lower to just above the start position, keeping tension on the muscles until the set is complete.
• Keep your elbows rigid without locking them at the top of the movement.
• Keep your torso stabilized.

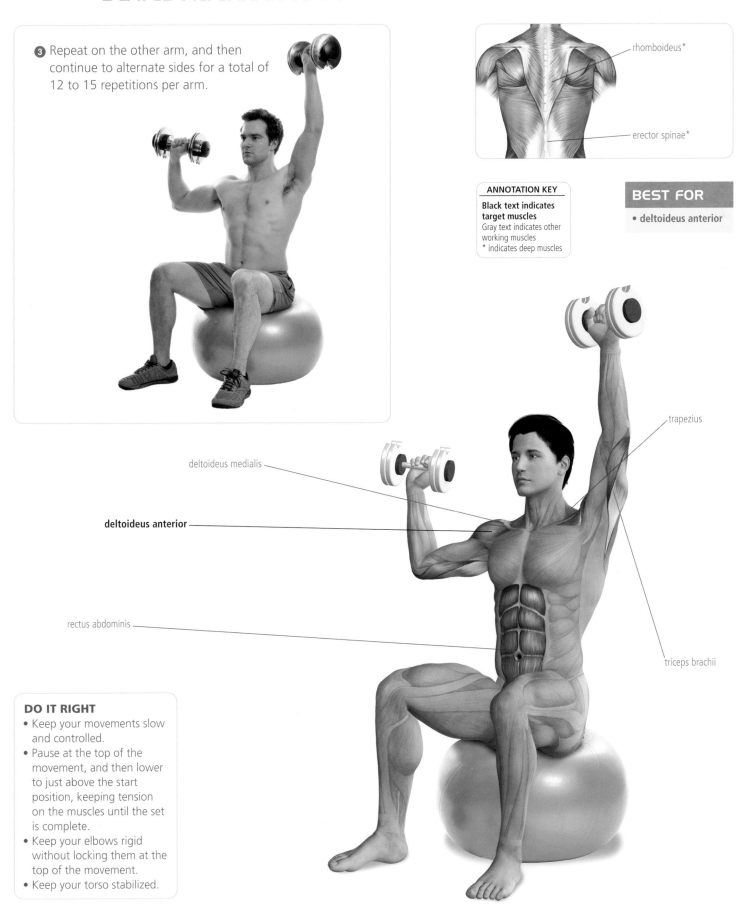

ONE-ARM SWISS BALL TRICEPS KICKBACK

1 Kneel with one arm resting on a Swiss ball. Grasping a dumbbell in the other hand, bend forward at the waist while keeping your upper arm tucked at your side.

AVOID
- Excessive speed.
- Hyperextending your arm.

TARGETS
- Triceps
- Core

LEVEL
- Beginner

BENEFITS
- Shapes and strengthens triceps
- Strengthens core

NOT ADVISABLE IF YOU HAVE . . .
- Knee issues
- Elbow pain

2 Extend the dumbbell back until your arm is fully extended and running parallel to the floor.

3 Return to the starting position and repeat for a total of 12 to 15 repetitions.

4 Switch sides and repeat on the other arm.

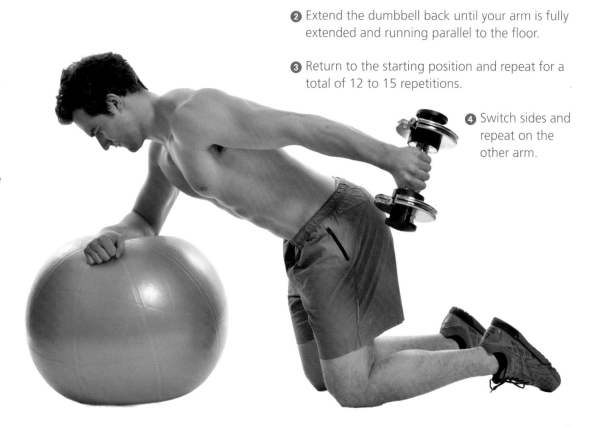

BEST FOR

- triceps brachii

DO IT RIGHT

- Keep your elbow tucked in at your side.
- Move through a complete range of motion.

MODIFICATION

Harder: Stand holding a pair of dumbbells and bend forward at the waist, keeping your elbows tucked into your sides. Follow steps 2 and 3.

ANNOTATION KEY

Black text indicates target muscles
Gray text indicates other working muscles
* indicates deep muscles

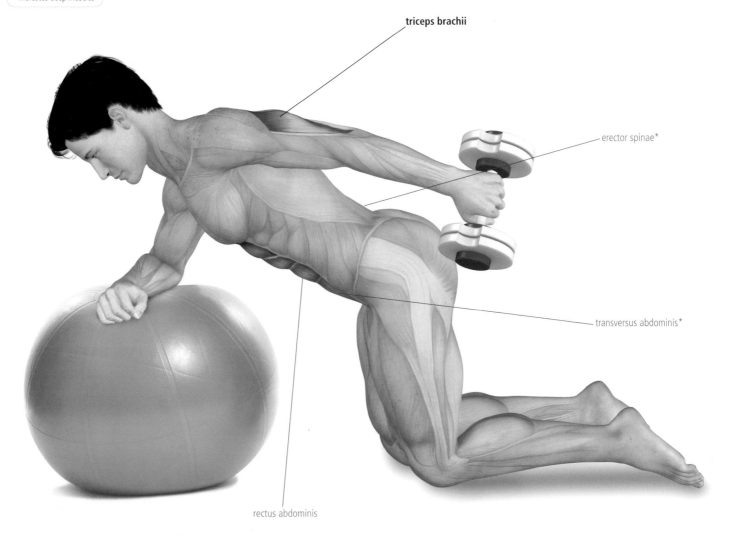

triceps brachii

erector spinae*

transversus abdominis*

rectus abdominis

DUMBBELL CALF RAISE

❶ Stand holding a pair of dumbbells at your sides with your toes placed on the edge of a raised platform.

❷ Rise up on your toes, contracting your calf muscles at the top, and then lower your heels back down past the edge of platform for a full stretch. Complete 12 to 15 repetitions.

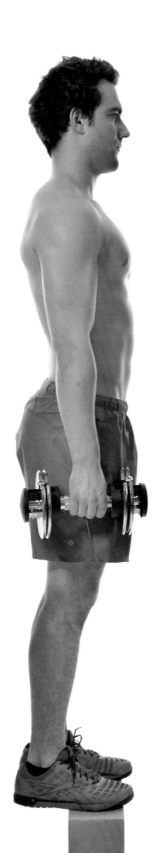

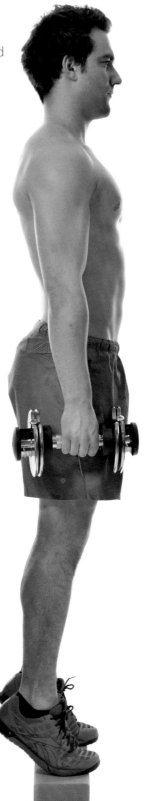

TARGETS
• Calves

LEVEL
• Beginner

BENEFITS
• Strengthens calf muscles

NOT ADVISABLE IF YOU HAVE . . .
• Ankle issues

BEST FOR
- gastrocnemius
- soleus

AVOID
- Excessive speed.
- Bouncy repetitions.

MODIFICATION
Similar level of difficulty:
Point your toes inward throughout the exercise.

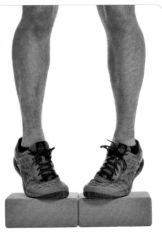

soleus

gastrocnemius

ANNOTATION KEY

Black text indicates target muscles
Gray text indicates other working muscles
* indicates deep muscles

DO IT RIGHT
- Maintain a full range of motion.
- Keep your toes pointed straight forward throughout the movement.
- Strongly contract your calf muscles with each repetition.

SWISS BALL FLYE

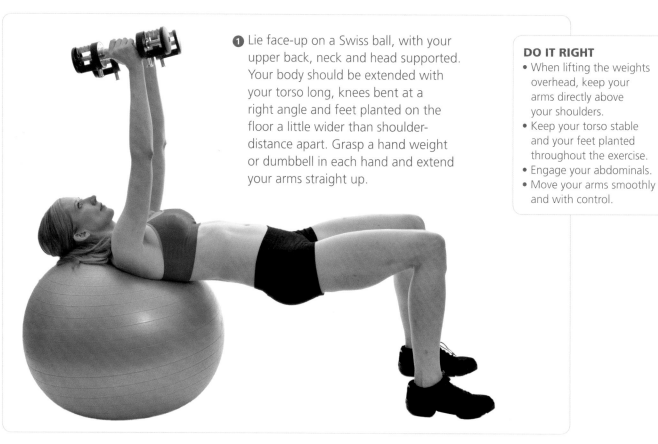

1 Lie face-up on a Swiss ball, with your upper back, neck and head supported. Your body should be extended with your torso long, knees bent at a right angle and feet planted on the floor a little wider than shoulder-distance apart. Grasp a hand weight or dumbbell in each hand and extend your arms straight up.

DO IT RIGHT
- When lifting the weights overhead, keep your arms directly above your shoulders.
- Keep your torso stable and your feet planted throughout the exercise.
- Engage your abdominals.
- Move your arms smoothly and with control.

TARGETS
- Chest

LEVEL
- Beginner

BENEFITS
- Strengthens and tones pectoral muscles

NOT ADVISABLE IF YOU HAVE . . .
- Shoulder issues

2 Keeping the rest of your body stable, bend your arms slightly as you stretch them out to the sides in a reverse hugging motion.

3 Return your arms to starting position. Repeat, completing 12 to 15 repetitions.

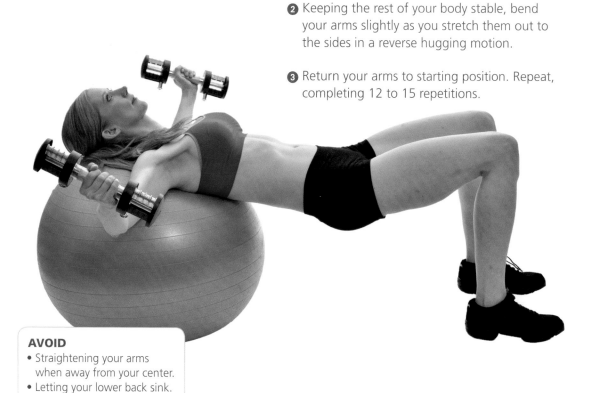

AVOID
- Straightening your arms when away from your center.
- Letting your lower back sink.

BEST FOR
- pectoralis major
- pectoralis minor

ANNOTATION KEY

Black text indicates target muscles
Gray text indicates other working muscles
* indicates deep muscles

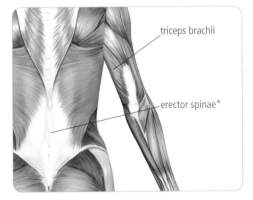

triceps brachii

erector spinae*

MODIFICATION

Similar level of difficulty: Instead of holding hand weights, loop a fitness band under your ball and grasp a handle in each hand. Keep your arms extended as you hold the strap taut throughout the exercise.

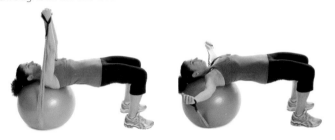

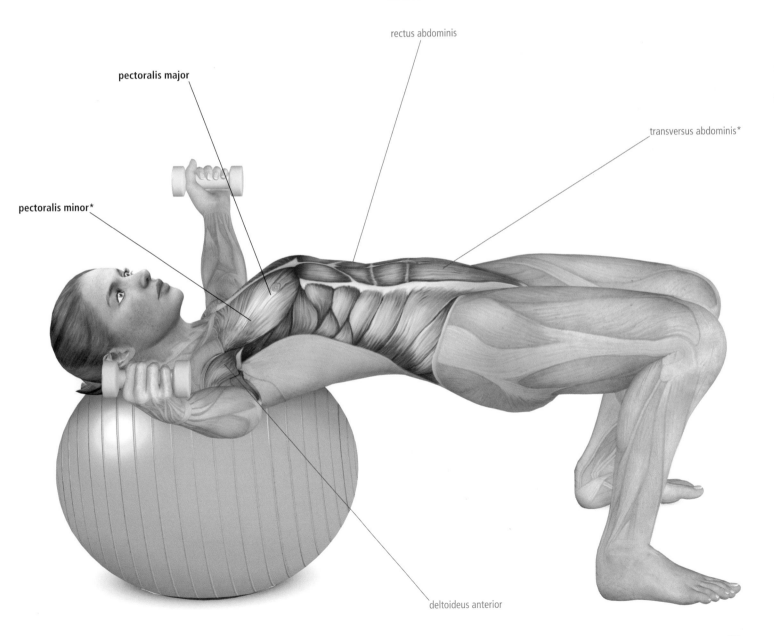

rectus abdominis

pectoralis major

transversus abdominis*

pectoralis minor*

deltoideus anterior

SWISS BALL REAR LATERAL RAISE

❶ Lie facedown on a Swiss ball with a pair of dumbbells at your sides, your palms facing inward and your legs spaced slightly apart for stability.

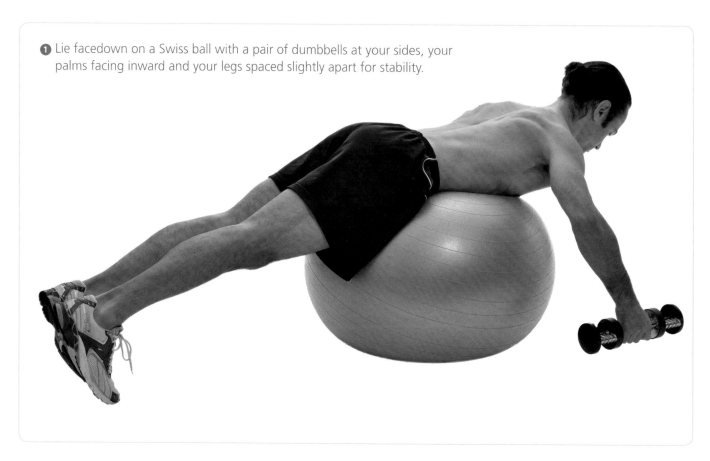

TARGETS
• Shoulders
• Upper back
• Chest

LEVEL
• Intermediate

BENEFITS
• Strengthens and builds the rear of the shoulders and upper back and shoulders
• Helps improve posture
• Stretches and tones chest muscles

NOT ADVISABLE IF YOU HAVE . . .
• Neck issues
• Lower-back pain

❷ Raise your arms directly out to the sides in a reverse hugging motion, bending your arms slightly.

❸ Lower your arms back to start position and repeat for 12 to 15 repetitions.

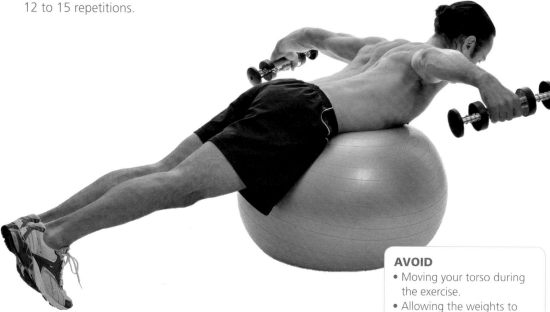

AVOID
• Moving your torso during the exercise.
• Allowing the weights to touch the floor.

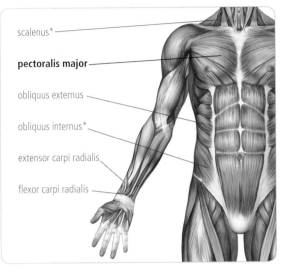

scalenus*

pectoralis major

obliquus externus

obliquus internus*

extensor carpi radialis

flexor carpi radialis

BEST FOR

- deltoideus posterior
- rhomboideus
- teres minor
- trapezius
- deltoideus medialis
- pectoralis major

ANNOTATION KEY

Black text indicates target muscles
Gray text indicates other working muscles
* indicates deep muscles

DO IT RIGHT

- Keep a slight bend in your elbows throughout the entire exercise.
- Raise your elbows as high as you can, so that they both reach the same height.

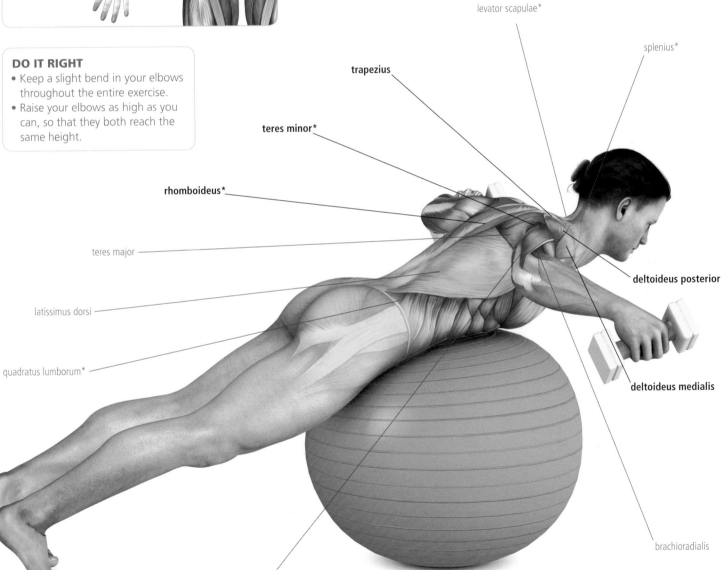

levator scapulae*

splenius*

trapezius

teres minor*

rhomboideus*

teres major

latissimus dorsi

quadratus lumborum*

deltoideus posterior

deltoideus medialis

brachioradialis

triceps brachii

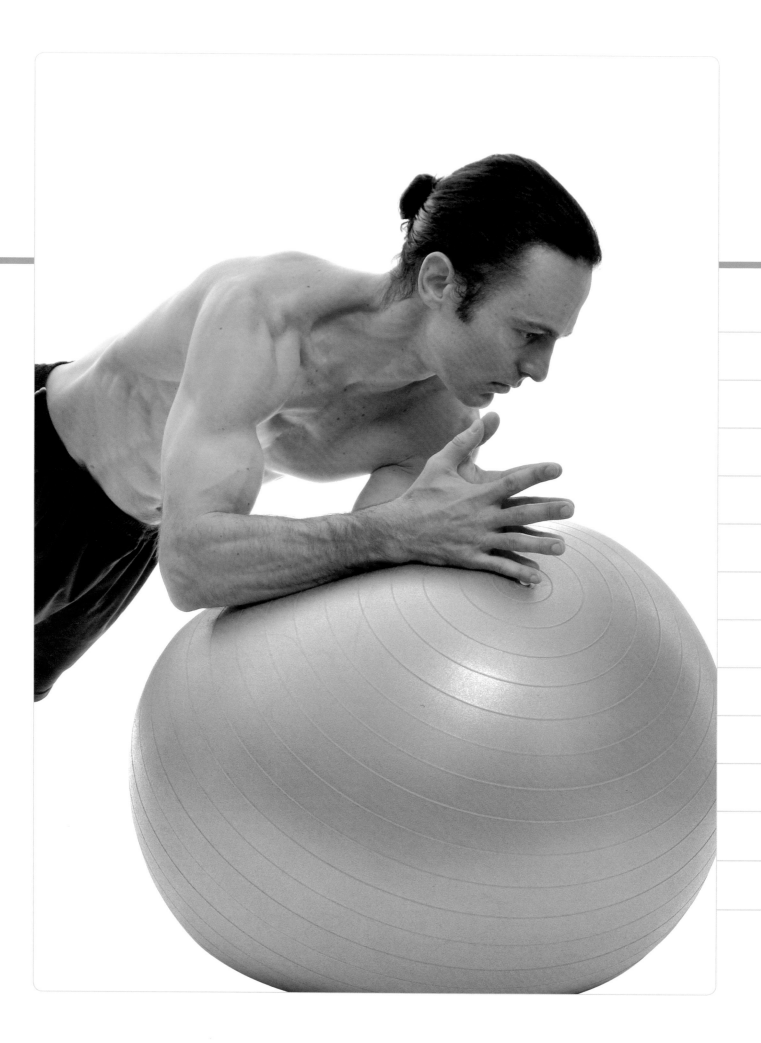

POSTURAL/CORE EXERCISES

Beyond the tight tummy most of us dream of showcasing lies the core, whose job is to support your spine. The core is composed of your pelvic and hip muscles, lower back and, yes, your abdominal muscles. The core provides support for all body movement, and improving your core strength will result in better posture, stability, alignment and more. A strong core also protects your vulnerable back, distributing the stress of weight-bearing, which will make everyday activities, from carrying groceries to sitting at a desk, easier.

Core training differs from that of traditional strength training in that instead of muscle isolation, here your are unifying or working groups of muscles together as a whole to complete a given coordinated movement.

KNEELING TO SEMI-KNEELING PROGRESSION

1 Kneel with your forehead on the floor and your arms running parallel to your lower legs and your palms facing upward. Curl up until your rear is sitting on your heels.

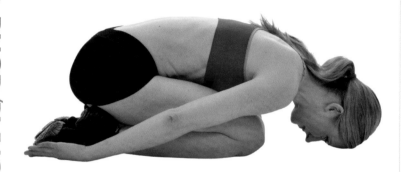

2 Begin slowly to rise to a kneeling position, elongating your spine as you rise.

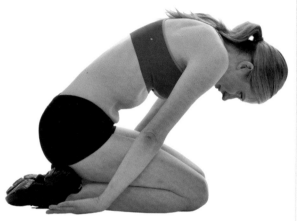

3 Continue to rise, extending your arms in front of you.

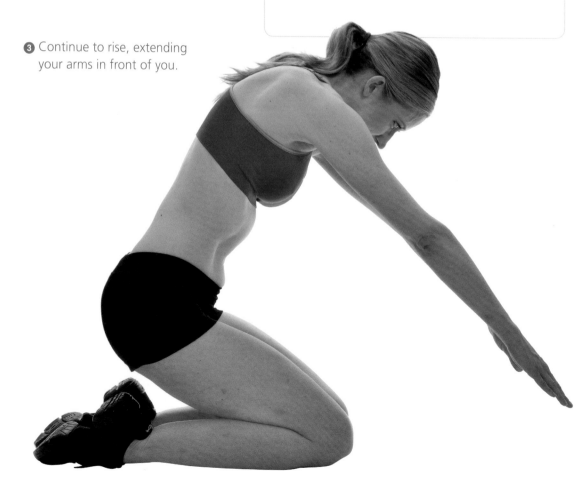

TARGETS
• Spine
• Core

LEVEL
• Beginner

BENEFITS
• Stabilizes the spine
• Strengthens and stabilizes core

NOT ADVISABLE IF YOU HAVE . . .
• Knee issues

4 Hold for 5 seconds, and repeat for a total of three repetitions.

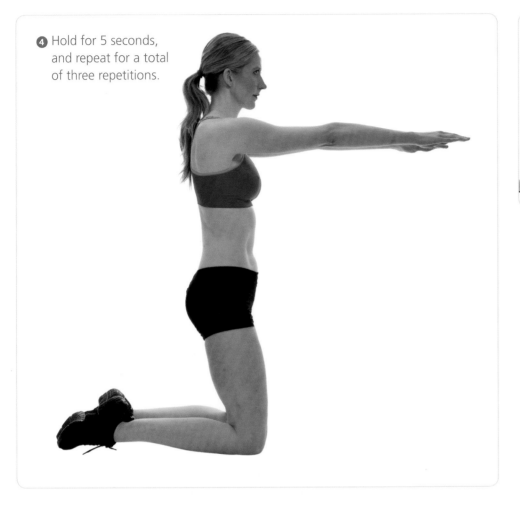

MODIFICATION
Harder: Perform the exercise holding a dumbbell in each hand.

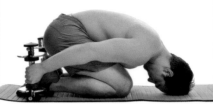

BEST FOR

• rectus femoris
• erector spinae

DO IT RIGHT
• Keep your pelvis braced throughout the exercise.

AVOID
• Excessive speed.

ANNOTATION KEY

Black text indicates target muscles
Gray text indicates other working muscles
* indicates deep muscles

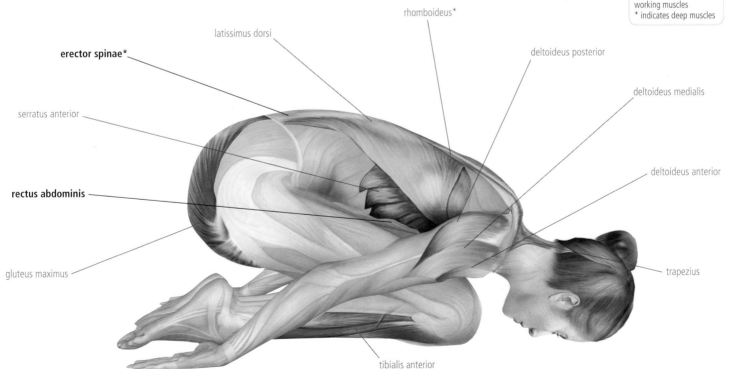

rhomboideus*

latissimus dorsi

erector spinae*

deltoideus posterior

deltoideus medialis

serratus anterior

rectus abdominis

deltoideus anterior

gluteus maximus

trapezius

tibialis anterior

PELVIC SIDE RAISE

1 Lie on your side with your knees bent and your feet behind you. Rest your top hand on your thigh, and brace your bottom forearm on the floor for support.

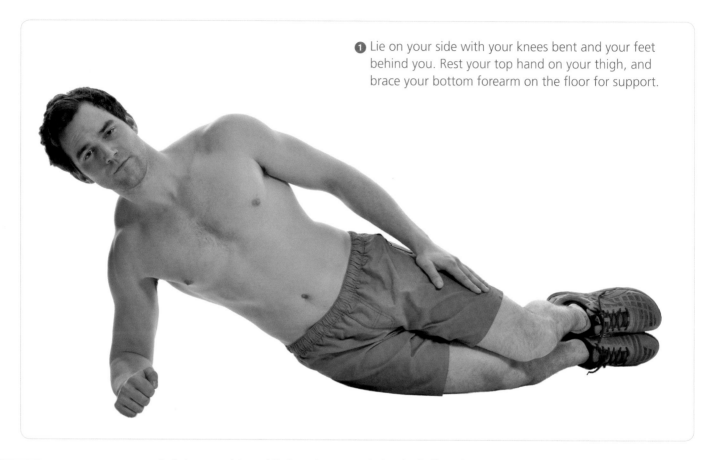

TARGETS
- Spine
- Core

LEVEL
- Beginner

BENEFITS
- Stabilizes the spine
- Strengthens and stabilizes core

NOT ADVISABLE IF YOU HAVE . . .
- Shoulder issues

2 Raise your hips while keeping your abdominals flexed or tensed, and hold for 5 seconds.

3 Switch positions, and repeat on the other side.

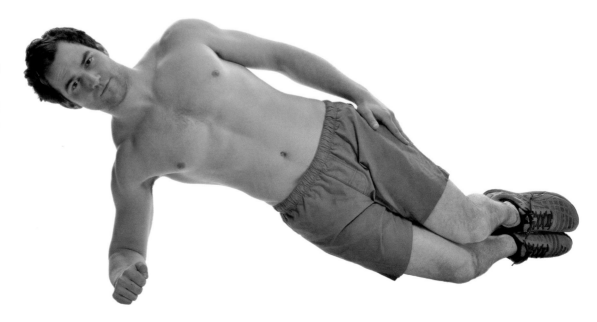

MODIFICATION

Harder: Keep your legs straight, with one on top of the other. Press into your forearm to lift your body into a side plank while raising your top arm toward the ceiling.

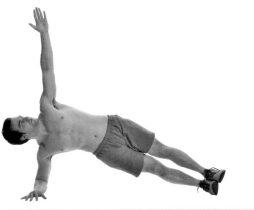

ANNOTATION KEY

Black text indicates target muscles
Gray text indicates other working muscles
* indicates deep muscles

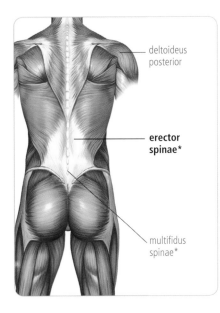

deltoideus posterior

erector spinae*

multifidus spinae*

BEST FOR

- erector spinae
- rectus abdominis
- transversus abdominis

DO IT RIGHT

- Keep your abdominal muscles tight throughout the exercise.

AVOID

- Placing too much strain on your shoulders.

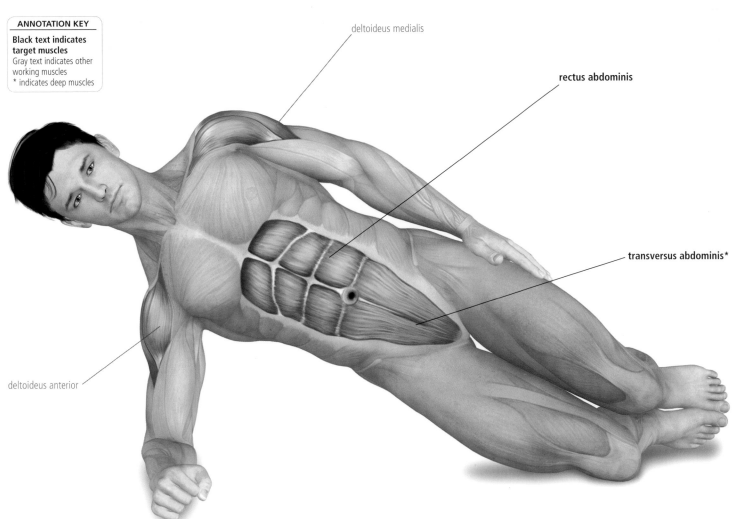

deltoideus medialis

rectus abdominis

transversus abdominis*

deltoideus anterior

TRUNK CURL

❶ Lie on your back with your legs bent and your fingers interlocked behind your head.

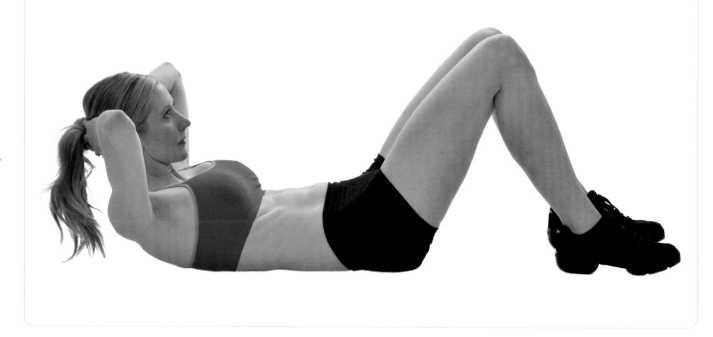

TARGETS
• Abdominals

LEVEL
• Beginner

BENEFITS
• Strengthens core muscles
• Increases abdominal endurance

NOT ADVISABLE IF YOU HAVE . . .
• Neck issues

❷ While keeping your abdominals flexed or tensed, slowly raise your shoulders toward your knees while keeping your heels pressed into the floor.

❸ Slowly lower back to the starting position, and repeat for 20 repetitions.

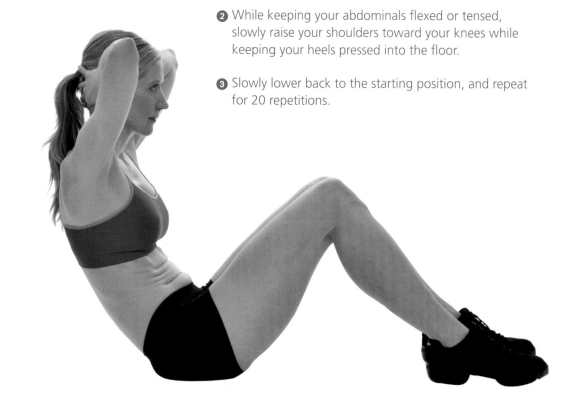

BEST FOR

- rectus abdominis
- transversus abdominis
- erector spinae
- sternohyoideus
- sternocleidomastoideus

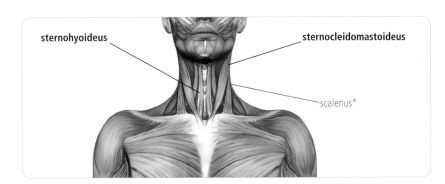

sternohyoideus

sternocleidomastoideus

scalenus*

DO IT RIGHT
- Lead with your abdominals, not your neck.

AVOID
- Excessive speed or using momentum to drive the movement.
- Allowing your feet to raise off the floor.
- Raising your torso too high.

ANNOTATION KEY

Black text indicates target muscles
Gray text indicates other working muscles
* indicates deep muscles

rectus abdominis

transversus abdominis*

obliquus externus

obliquus internus*

latissimus dorsi

erector spinae*

tensor fasciae latae

REVERSE TRUNK CURL

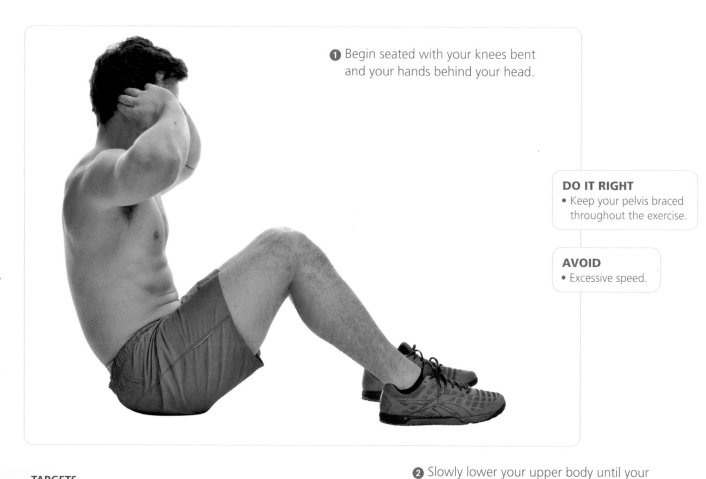

1 Begin seated with your knees bent and your hands behind your head.

DO IT RIGHT
• Keep your pelvis braced throughout the exercise.

AVOID
• Excessive speed.

TARGETS
• Abdominals

LEVEL
• Beginner

BENEFITS
• Strengthens core muscles
• Increases abdominal endurance

NOT ADVISABLE IF YOU HAVE . . .
• Neck issues

2 Slowly lower your upper body until your shoulder blades are touching the floor.

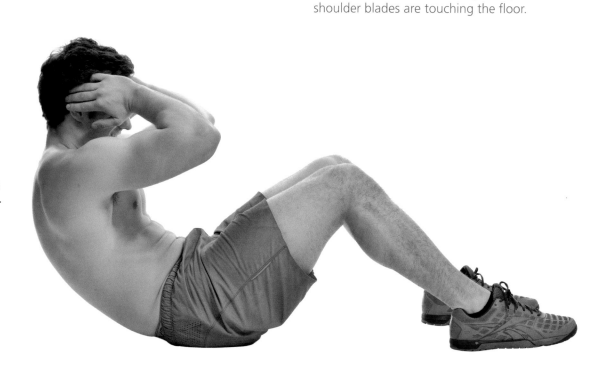

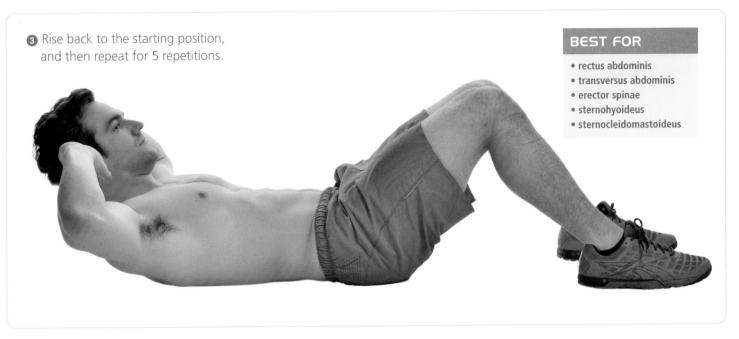

❸ Rise back to the starting position, and then repeat for 5 repetitions.

BEST FOR

- rectus abdominis
- transversus abdominis
- erector spinae
- sternohyoideus
- sternocleidomastoideus

ANNOTATION KEY

Black text indicates target muscles
Gray text indicates other working muscles
* indicates deep muscles

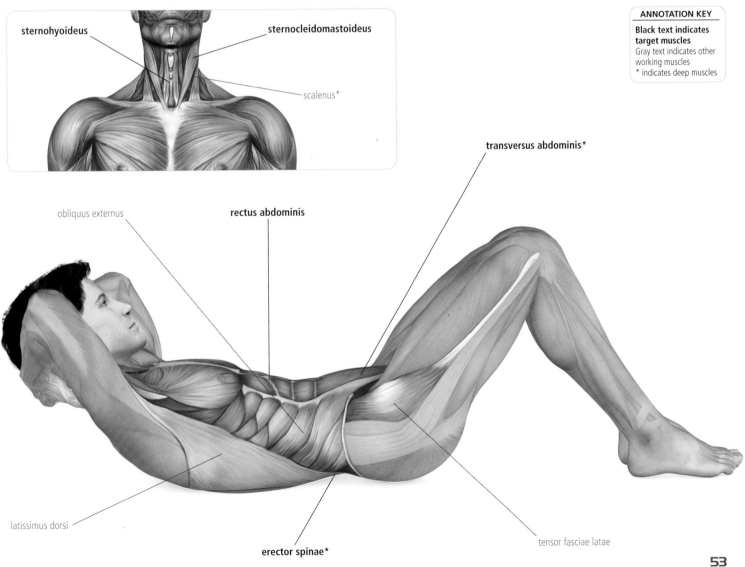

sternohyoideus

sternocleidomastoideus

scalenus*

transversus abdominis*

obliquus externus

rectus abdominis

latissimus dorsi

erector spinae*

tensor fasciae latae

WALL SQUAT

① Stand with your back pressed against a wall and your feet spaced shoulder-width apart. Your feet should be that same distance from the wall.

BEST FOR

- rectus femoris
- vastus lateralis
- vastus intermedius
- vastus medialis
- gluteus maximus
- biceps femoris
- semitendinosus
- semimembranosus

DO IT RIGHT
- Push through your heels to drive the movement.
- Be sure to squat until your thighs are parallel to the floor.

② Bend at the knees, squatting toward the floor while keeping your lower back pressed against the wall.

③ Push through your heels to rise. Complete 12 to 15 repetitions.

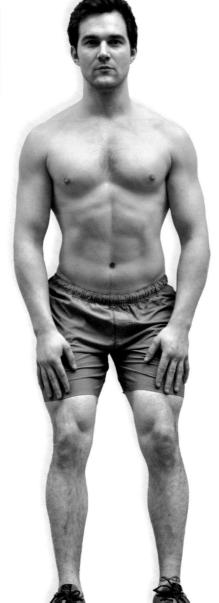

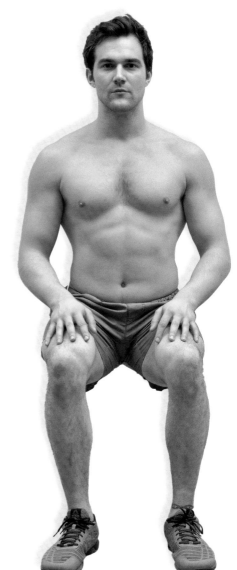

TARGETS
- Thighs
- Glutes
- Core

LEVEL
- Beginner

BENEFITS
- Strengthens quadriceps, buttocks and core

NOT ADVISABLE IF YOU HAVE . . .
- Knee issues

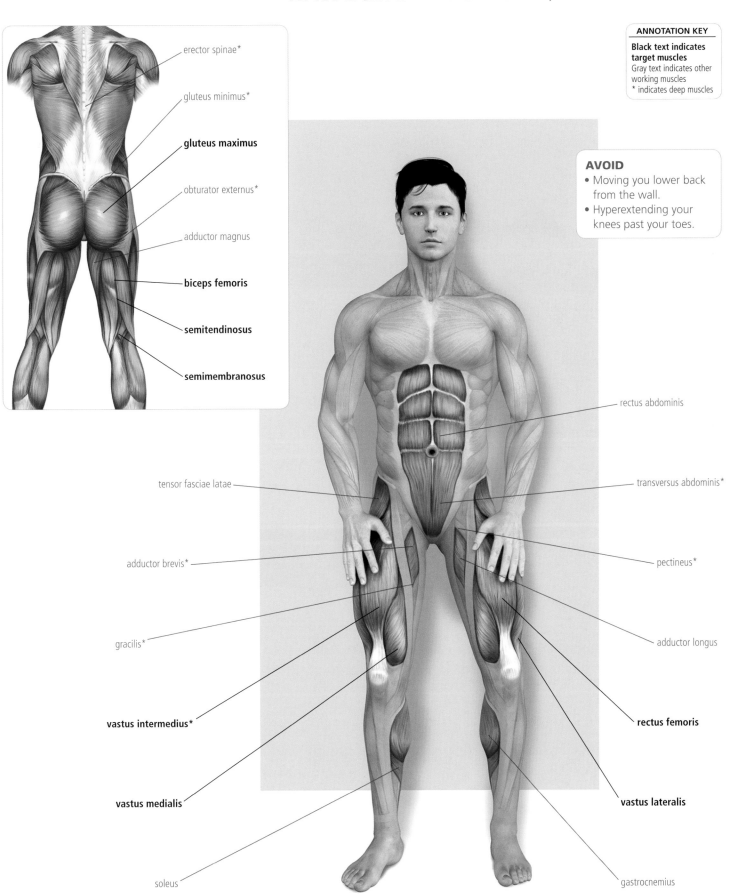

ANNOTATION KEY

Black text indicates target muscles
Gray text indicates other working muscles
* indicates deep muscles

erector spinae*

gluteus minimus*

gluteus maximus

obturator externus*

adductor magnus

biceps femoris

semitendinosus

semimembranosus

AVOID
• Moving you lower back from the wall.
• Hyperextending your knees past your toes.

rectus abdominis

tensor fasciae latae

transversus abdominis*

adductor brevis*

pectineus*

gracilis*

adductor longus

vastus intermedius*

rectus femoris

vastus medialis

vastus lateralis

soleus

gastrocnemius

PILATES X

1 Lie on your stomach with both your legs and arms fully extended forming an X.

BEST FOR

- erector spinae
- rectus abdominis
- gluteus maximus
- deltoideus anterior
- deltoideus medialis
- deltoideus posterior

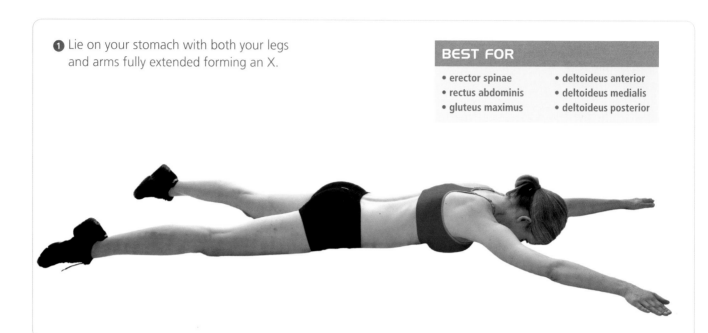

2 Inhale as you simultaneously lift your legs and arms off the floor, tightening your abdominal muscles as you lift.

TARGETS
- Core
- Glutes
- Shoulders
- Spine

LEVEL
- Beginner

BENEFITS
- Strengthens core
- Helps improve posture

NOT ADVISABLE IF YOU HAVE . . .
- Lower-back pain

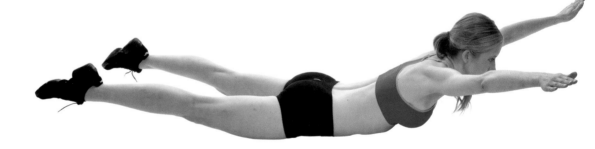

3 Exhale while drawing your legs together and bend your elbows toward your waist.

4 Repeat for 10 to 12 repetitions.

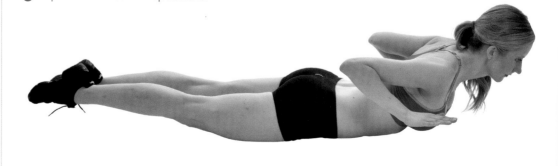

DO IT RIGHT
- Extend your limbs as long as possible.
- Tightly squeeze your glutes, and draw your navel in toward your spine throughout the exercise.

AVOID
- Holding your breath.
- Excessive speed.
- Allowing your shoulders to lift toward your ears.

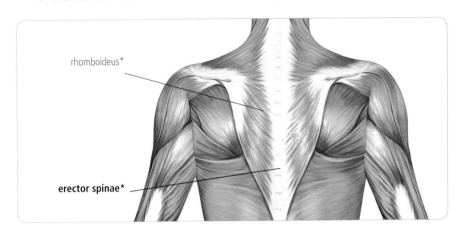

rhomboideus*

erector spinae*

ANNOTATION KEY

Black text indicates target muscles
Gray text indicates other working muscles
* indicates deep muscles

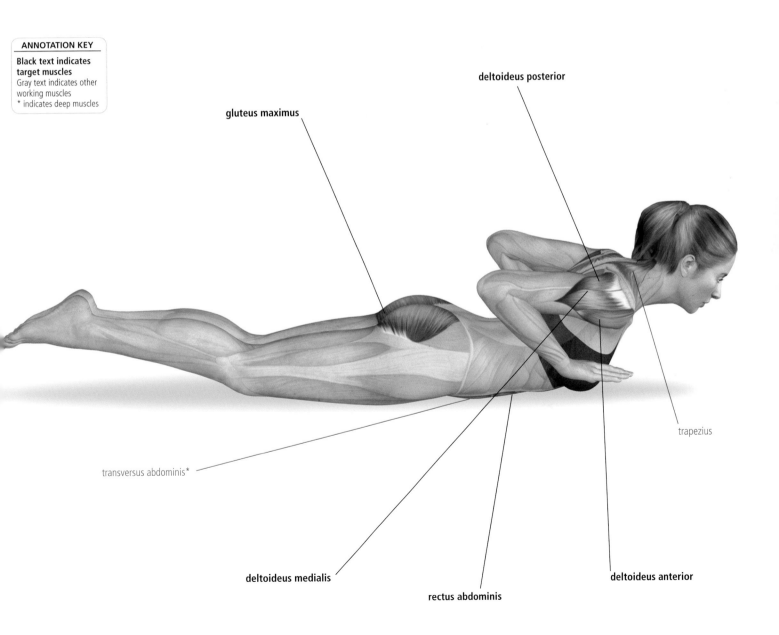

deltoideus posterior

gluteus maximus

trapezius

transversus abdominis*

deltoideus medialis

rectus abdominis

deltoideus anterior

SWISS BALL CIRCLES

1 Begin in a plank position with your feet hip-width apart on the floor and your forearms planted on a Swiss ball. Elongate your spine, and support your weight with your toes.

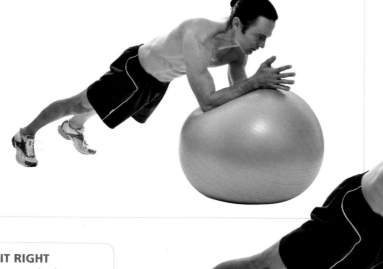

DO IT RIGHT
- Keep your body one straight line throughout the movement.

TARGETS
- Core
- Spine

LEVEL
- Intermediate

BENEFITS
- Strengthens and stabilizes core

NOT ADVISABLE IF YOU HAVE . . .
- Shoulder issues
- Severe lower-back pain

2 Roll toward all four points of direction, tracing a circle with your elbows, pressing your forearms into the ball during the entire movement. Return to center. A complete circle is one repetition.

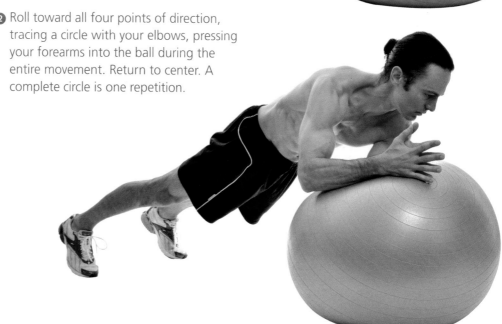

3 Complete 8 to 10 reps, and then reverse direction.

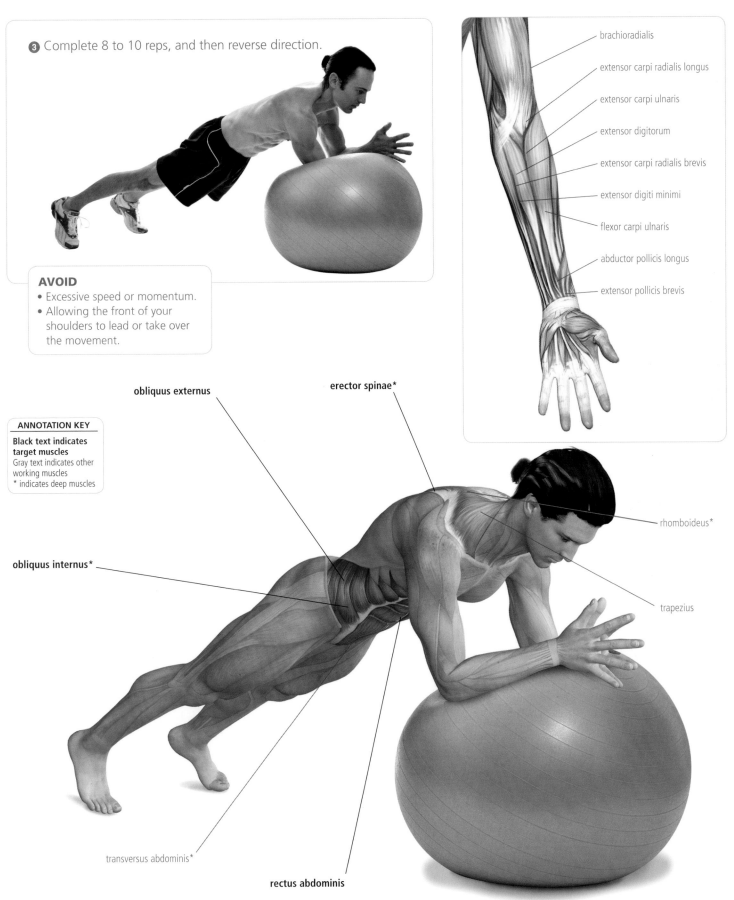

AVOID
- Excessive speed or momentum.
- Allowing the front of your shoulders to lead or take over the movement.

brachioradialis

extensor carpi radialis longus

extensor carpi ulnaris

extensor digitorum

extensor carpi radialis brevis

extensor digiti minimi

flexor carpi ulnaris

abductor pollicis longus

extensor pollicis brevis

obliquus externus

erector spinae*

ANNOTATION KEY

Black text indicates target muscles
Gray text indicates other working muscles
* indicates deep muscles

rhomboideus*

obliquus internus*

trapezius

transversus abdominis*

rectus abdominis

SWISS BALL W

❶ Lie facedown on a Swiss ball with your back flat, your chest off the ball, and your legs elongated. Bend your elbows, keeping them close to your sides.

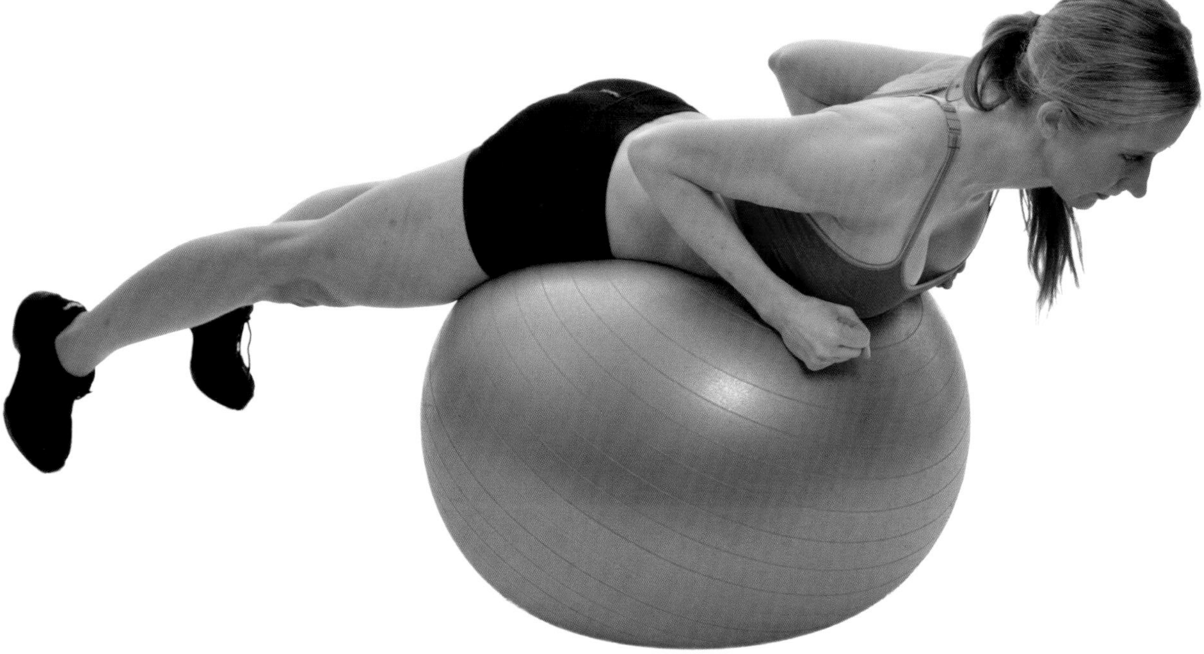

TARGETS
• Shoulders
• Core

LEVEL
• Intermediate

BENEFITS
• Strengthens the rear of the shoulders
• Stabilizes core
• Helps improve posture

NOT ADVISABLE IF YOU HAVE . . .
• Shoulder issues
• Severe lower-back pain

❷ Keeping your elbows bent, squeeze your shoulder blades together as you raise your upper arms. Your arms will form a W at the top of the movement.

❸ Hold briefly, and then slowly lower to the starting position. Repeat for 12 to 15 repetitions.

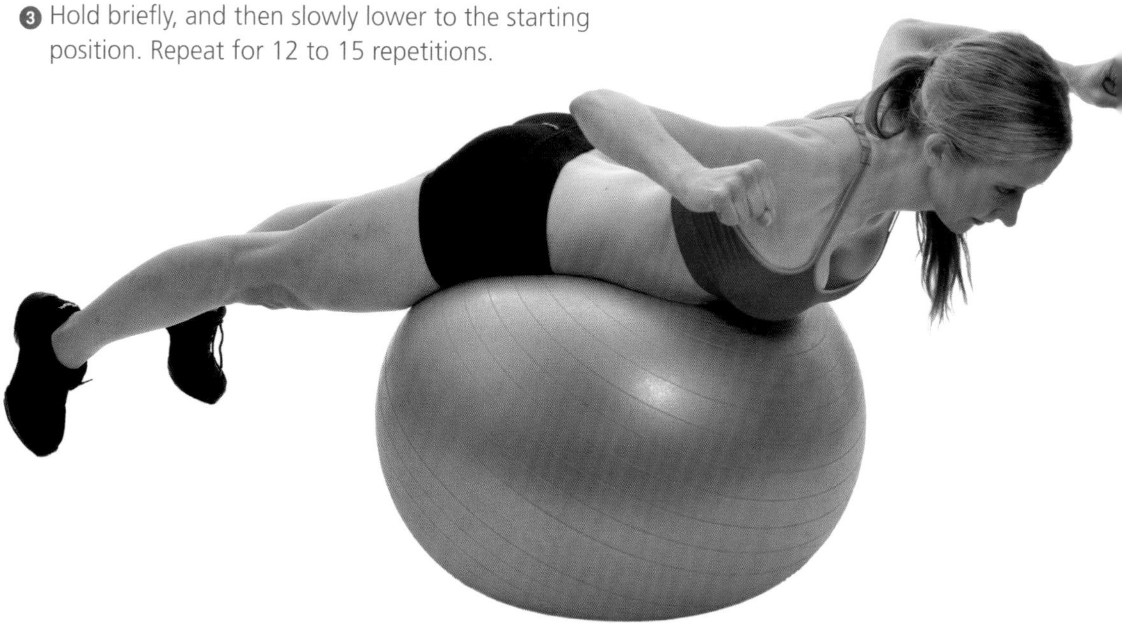

DO IT RIGHT
- Keep our arms bent throughout the movement.
- Use a reverse hugging motion.

AVOID
- Excessive speed or momentum.

BEST FOR
- deltoideus posterior

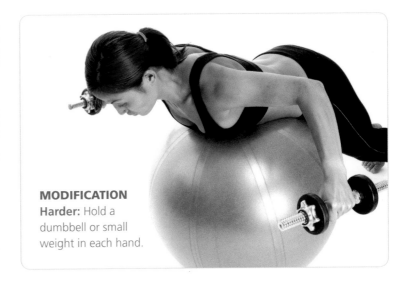

MODIFICATION
Harder: Hold a dumbbell or small weight in each hand.

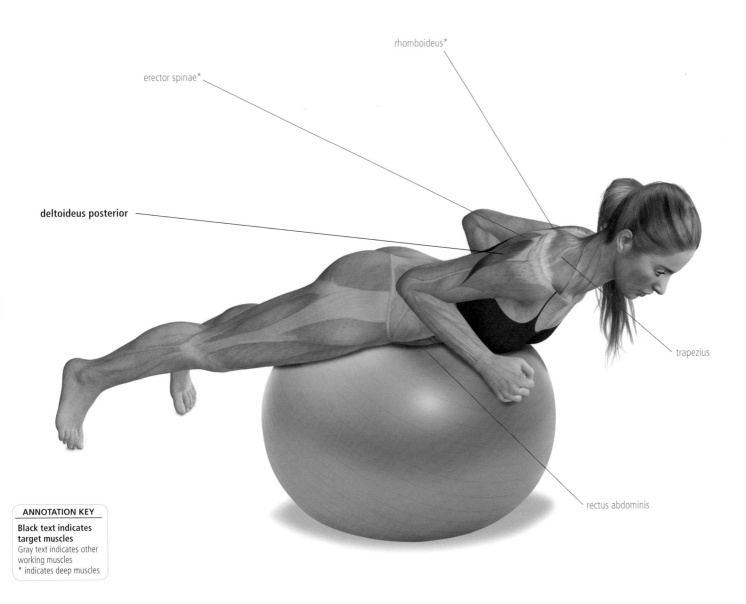

rhomboideus*

erector spinae*

deltoideus posterior

trapezius

rectus abdominis

ANNOTATION KEY

Black text indicates target muscles
Gray text indicates other working muscles
* indicates deep muscles

SWISS BALL LUMBAR ROTATION

❶ Lie on your back, with your arms extended out to your sides. Place your legs on a Swiss ball, with your glutes close to the ball.

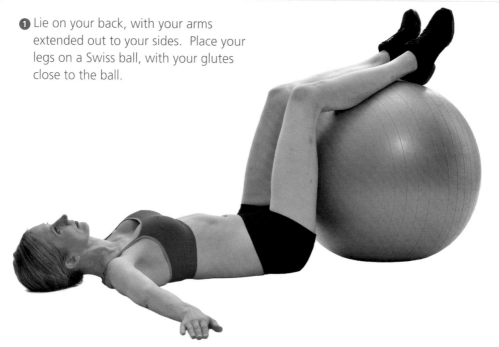

AVOID
• Swinging your legs too quickly; instead, try to keep the movement smooth and controlled.

❷ Brace your abs, and lower your legs to one side, as close to the floor as you can possibly go without raising your shoulders off the floor.

TARGETS
• Lower back
• Obliques

LEVEL
• Beginner

BENEFITS
• Helps to strengthen and tone abs
• Stabilizes core

NOT ADVISABLE IF YOU HAVE . . .
• Lower-back issues

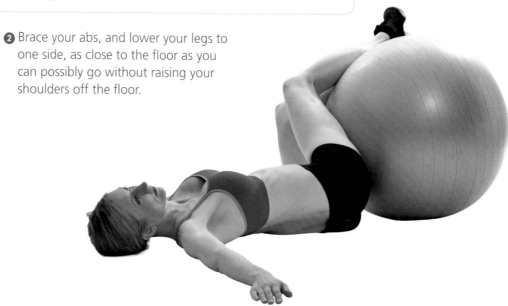

MODIFICATION
Easier: Begin with your legs lifted and bent at a 90-degree angle. Try to keep your upper body as stable as possible as you perform the crossover without the ball, alternating sides.

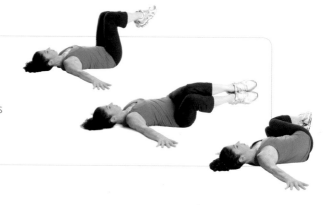

3 Return to the starting position, and then repeat on the other side. Work up to completing 20 in each direction.

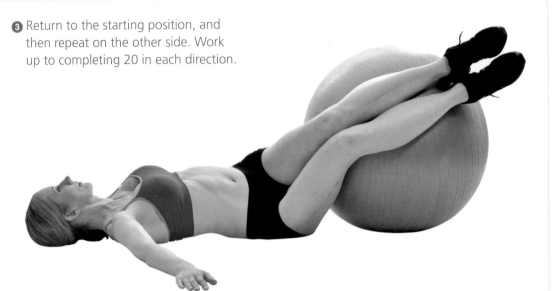

BEST FOR

- erector spinae
- rectus abdominis
- obliquus externus
- obliquus internus

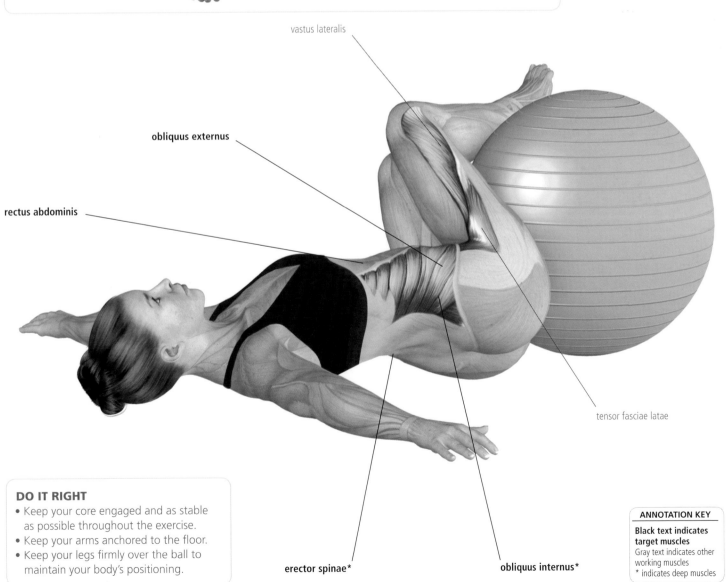

vastus lateralis

obliquus externus

rectus abdominis

tensor fasciae latae

erector spinae*

obliquus internus*

DO IT RIGHT

- Keep your core engaged and as stable as possible throughout the exercise.
- Keep your arms anchored to the floor.
- Keep your legs firmly over the ball to maintain your body's positioning.

ANNOTATION KEY

Black text indicates target muscles
Gray text indicates other working muscles
* indicates deep muscles

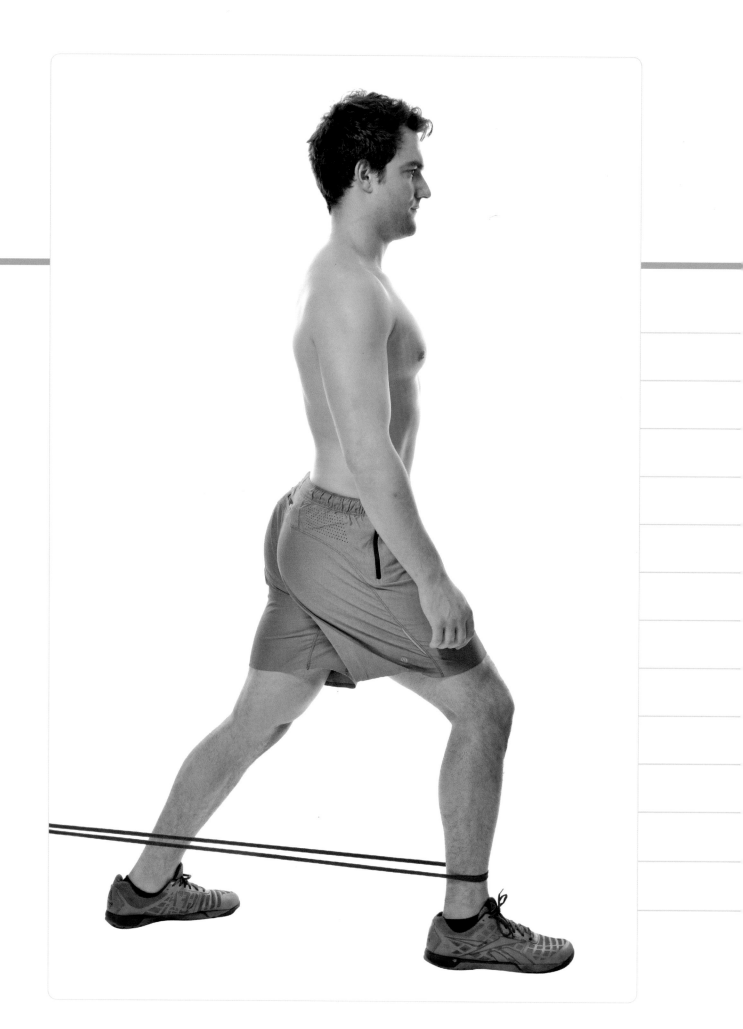

MOBILITY EXERCISES

If the term *flexibility* equates to the range of motion around a given joint,

then *mobility* refers to how well you can move through a given range of

motion. You must incorporate mobility training into your current fitness

regimen, identifying and resolving movement limitations that can decrease

your performance and/or lead to injury. Mobility training calls for exercises

that mainly use your own body weight, thoroughly warming up a given muscle

and its target pathway. For a modality that can take mere minutes to complete

per day, the rewards are well worth the time spent, resulting in your ability to

move through life both pain and injury free.

COUCH STRETCH

❶ Begin on the floor with your back leg bent and your shin and foot placed against the wall and the other leg forward with your foot flat.

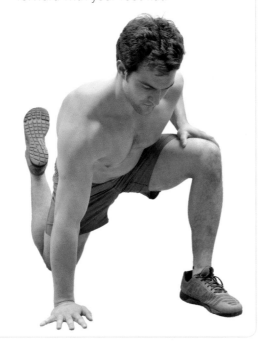

❷ Arch and relax your back, holding the position for one to two minutes.

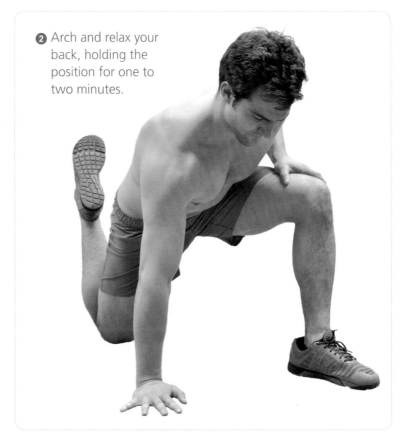

TARGETS
- Glutes
- Quadriceps
- Hip flexors

LEVEL
- Beginner

BENEFITS
- Increases the mobility and range of motion of ankles, knees and hips

NOT ADVISABLE IF YOU HAVE . . .
- Knee issues

BEST FOR
- **gluteus maximus**
- **rectus femoris**
- **vastus lateralis**
- **vastus intermedius**
- **vastus medialis**
- **iliopsoas**
- **sartorius**

❷ Switch sides, and then repeat on the other leg.

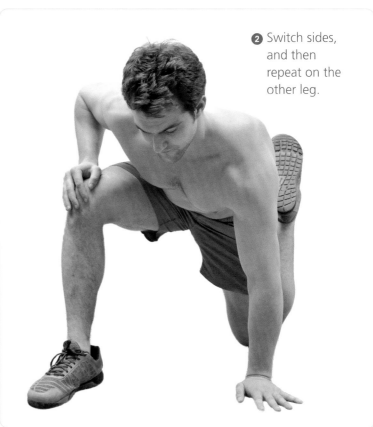

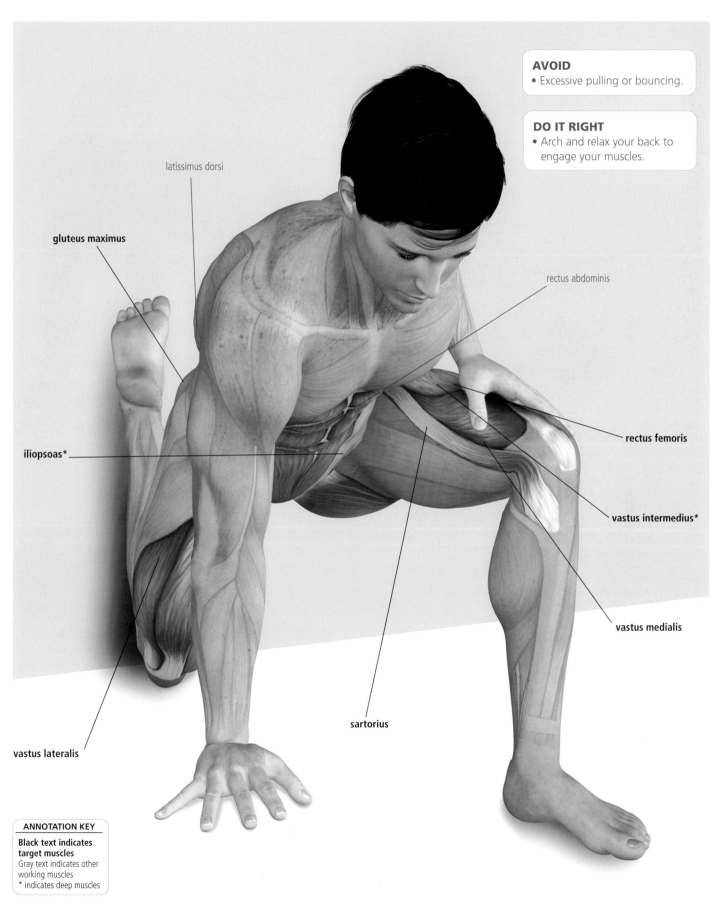

AVOID
• Excessive pulling or bouncing.

DO IT RIGHT
• Arch and relax your back to engage your muscles.

latissimus dorsi

gluteus maximus

rectus abdominis

iliopsoas*

rectus femoris

vastus intermedius*

vastus medialis

sartorius

vastus lateralis

ANNOTATION KEY

Black text indicates target muscles
Gray text indicates other working muscles
* indicates deep muscles

POSTERIOR HIP MOBILIZATION

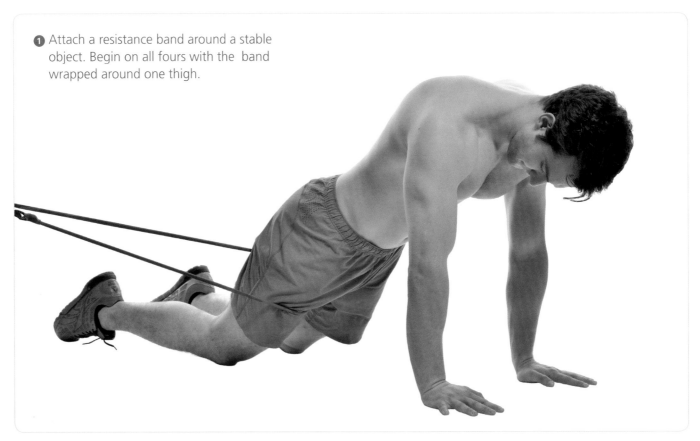

① Attach a resistance band around a stable object. Begin on all fours with the band wrapped around one thigh.

TARGETS
• Hips

LEVEL
• Beginner

BENEFITS
• Improves hip mobility and flexion

NOT ADVISABLE IF YOU HAVE . . .
• Knee issues

② Using the band's tension, swing your hip backward.

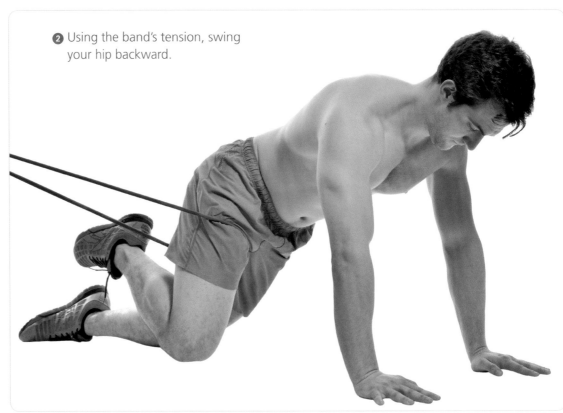

❸ Swing your hip forward, and then continue swinging backward and forward for one to two minutes. Switch sides, and repeat on the other leg.

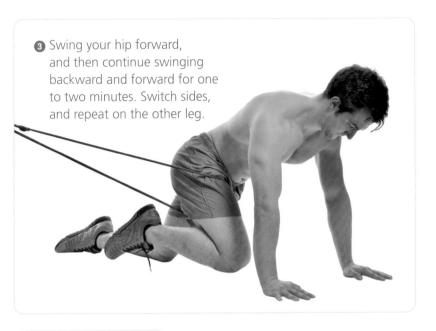

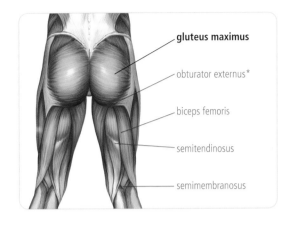

- gluteus maximus
- obturator externus*
- biceps femoris
- semitendinosus
- semimembranosus

ANNOTATION KEY

Black text indicates target muscles
Gray text indicates other working muscles
* indicates deep muscles

BEST FOR

- iliopsoas
- sartorius
- rectus femoris
- vastus lateralis
- vastus intermedius
- vastus medialis
- gluteus maximus

AVOID
- Excessive pulling against the band.
- Using momentum to drive the movement.

DO IT RIGHT
- Gently swing your hip against the band's resistance.

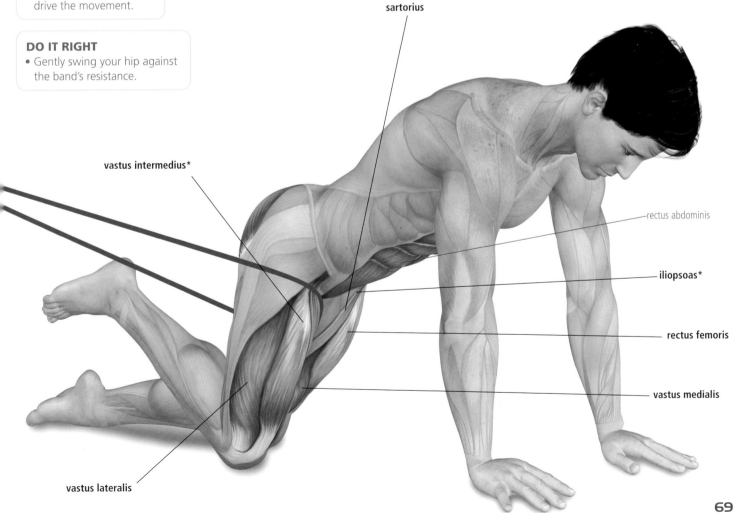

sartorius

vastus intermedius*

rectus abdominis

iliopsoas*

rectus femoris

vastus medialis

vastus lateralis

SQUAT TEST

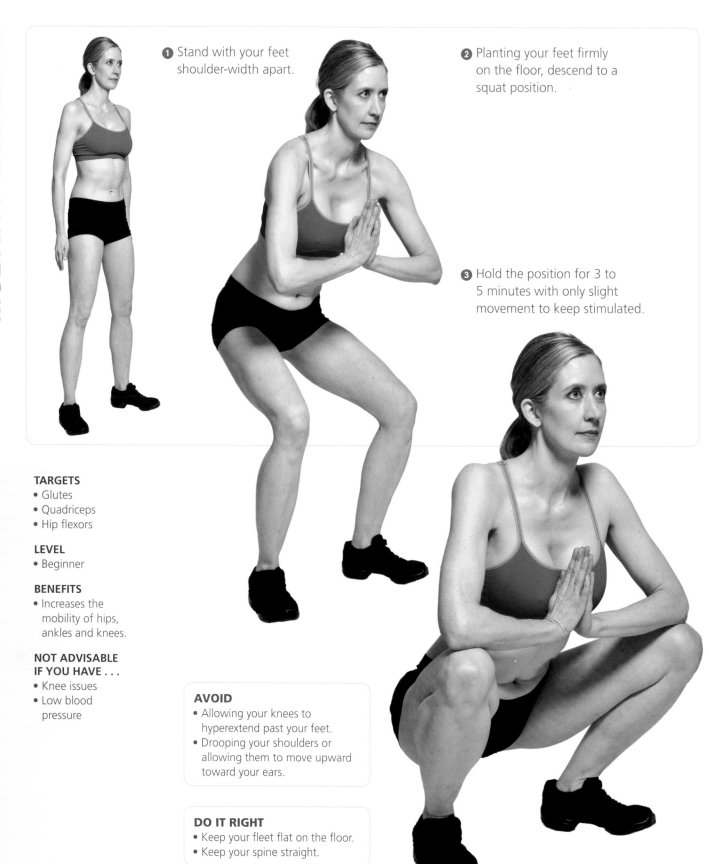

❶ Stand with your feet shoulder-width apart.

❷ Planting your feet firmly on the floor, descend to a squat position.

❸ Hold the position for 3 to 5 minutes with only slight movement to keep stimulated.

TARGETS
- Glutes
- Quadriceps
- Hip flexors

LEVEL
- Beginner

BENEFITS
- Increases the mobility of hips, ankles and knees.

NOT ADVISABLE IF YOU HAVE . . .
- Knee issues
- Low blood pressure

AVOID
- Allowing your knees to hyperextend past your feet.
- Drooping your shoulders or allowing them to move upward toward your ears.

DO IT RIGHT
- Keep your fleet flat on the floor.
- Keep your spine straight.

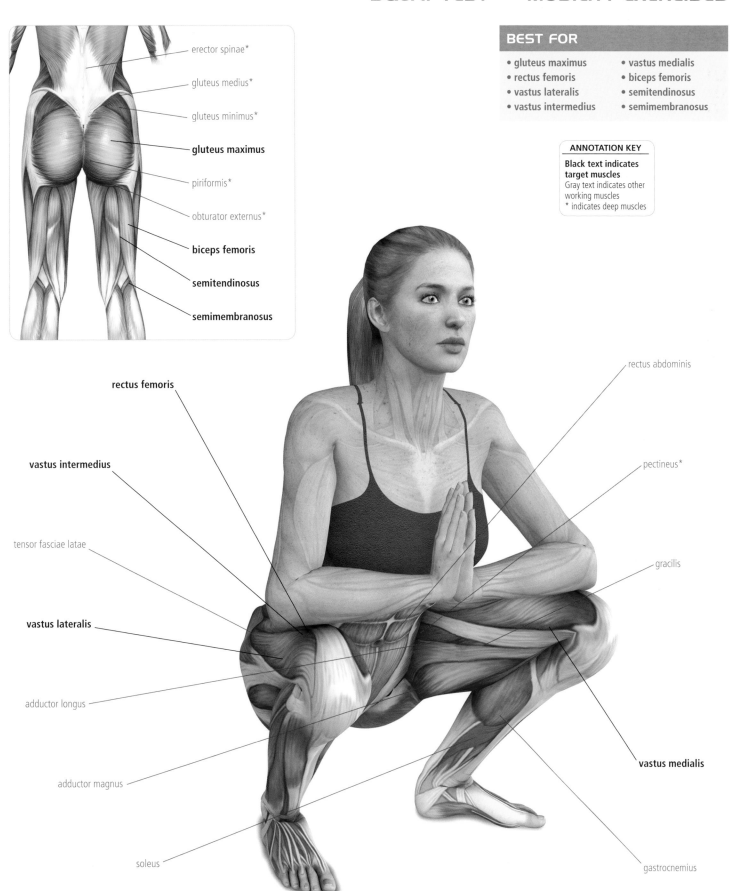

erector spinae*

gluteus medius*

gluteus minimus*

gluteus maximus

piriformis*

obturator externus*

biceps femoris

semitendinosus

semimembranosus

BEST FOR

- gluteus maximus
- rectus femoris
- vastus lateralis
- vastus intermedius
- vastus medialis
- biceps femoris
- semitendinosus
- semimembranosus

ANNOTATION KEY

Black text indicates target muscles
Gray text indicates other working muscles
* indicates deep muscles

rectus femoris

vastus intermedius

tensor fasciae latae

vastus lateralis

adductor longus

adductor magnus

soleus

rectus abdominis

pectineus*

gracilis

vastus medialis

gastrocnemius

ANTERIOR HIP MOBILIZATION

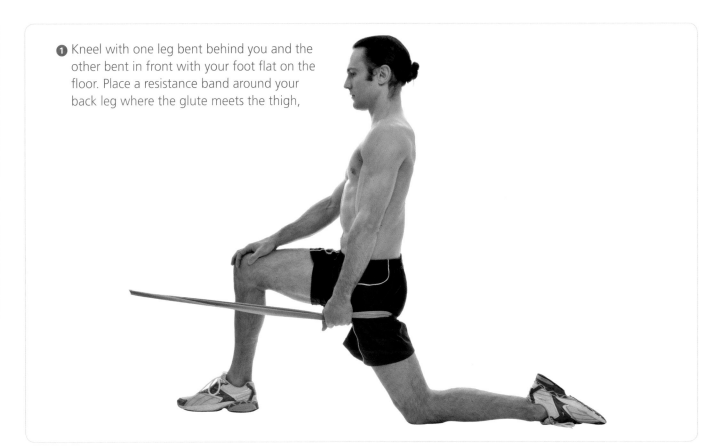

❶ Kneel with one leg bent behind you and the other bent in front with your foot flat on the floor. Place a resistance band around your back leg where the glute meets the thigh,

TARGETS
• Hips

LEVEL
• Beginner

BENEFITS
• Improves hip
  mobility
• Loosens tight
  hip flexors

**NOT ADVISABLE
IF YOU HAVE . . .**
• Knee issues

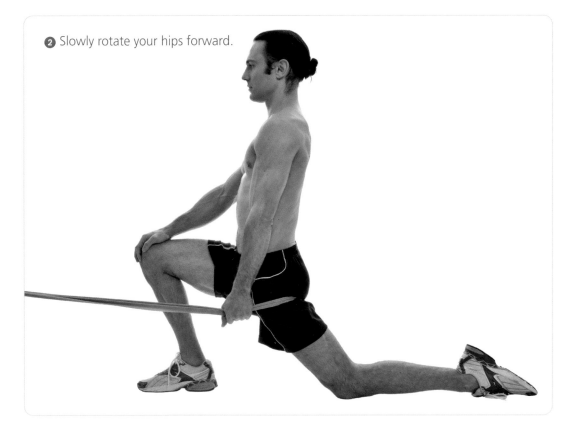

❷ Slowly rotate your hips forward.

❸ Continue to rotate your hips forward and back for 1 to 2 minutes. Switch sides, and repeat on the other hip.

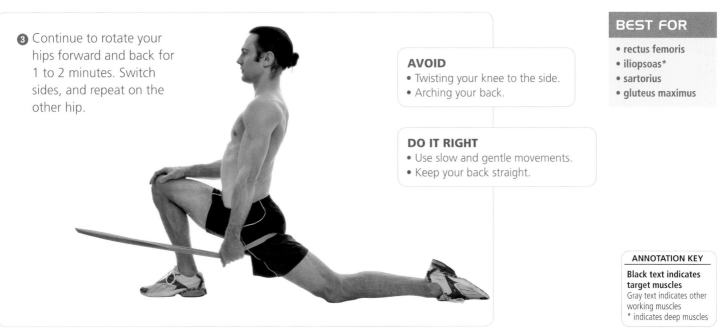

BEST FOR
- **rectus femoris**
- **iliopsoas***
- **sartorius**
- **gluteus maximus**

AVOID
- Twisting your knee to the side.
- Arching your back.

DO IT RIGHT
- Use slow and gentle movements.
- Keep your back straight.

ANNOTATION KEY
Black text indicates target muscles
Gray text indicates other working muscles
* indicates deep muscles

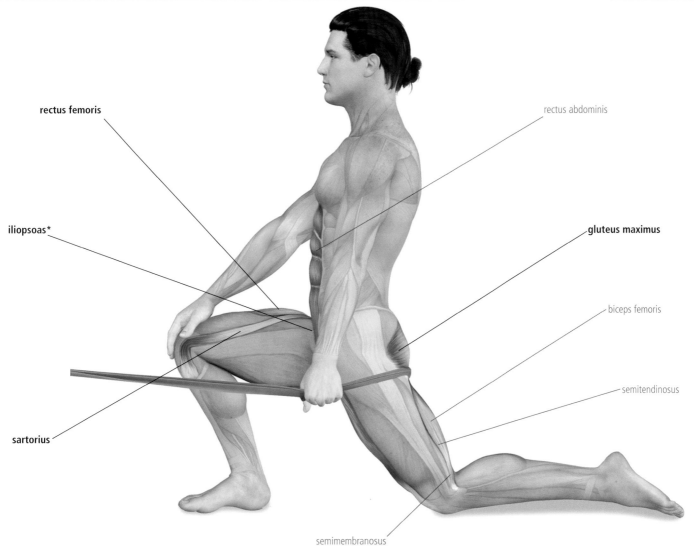

rectus femoris

rectus abdominis

iliopsoas*

gluteus maximus

biceps femoris

sartorius

semitendinosus

semimembranosus

ANKLE DORSIFLEXION

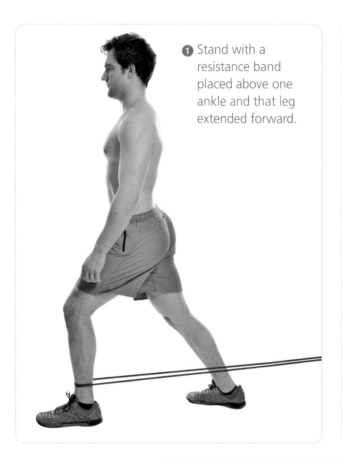

1 Stand with a resistance band placed above one ankle and that leg extended forward.

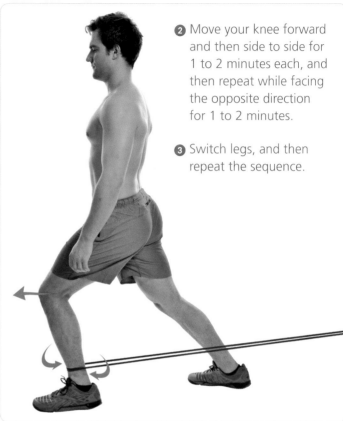

2 Move your knee forward and then side to side for 1 to 2 minutes each, and then repeat while facing the opposite direction for 1 to 2 minutes.

3 Switch legs, and then repeat the sequence.

TARGETS
• Ankles

LEVEL
• Beginner

BENEFITS
• Improves ankle mobility

NOT ADVISABLE IF YOU HAVE . . .
• Knee pain

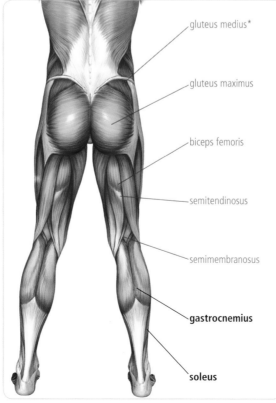

gluteus medius*

gluteus maximus

biceps femoris

semitendinosus

semimembranosus

gastrocnemius

soleus

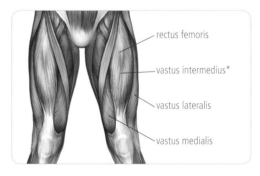

rectus femoris

vastus intermedius*

vastus lateralis

vastus medialis

AVOID
• Using momentum to drive the movement.

DO IT RIGHT
• Use slow and gentle movements.

ANNOTATION KEY

Black text indicates target muscles
Gray text indicates other working muscles
* indicates deep muscles

BEST FOR
• soleus
• gastrocnemius

EXTERNAL ROTATION SHOULDER EXTENSION

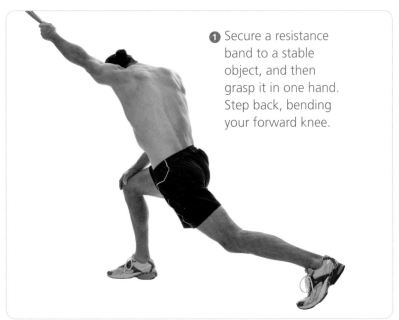

1 Secure a resistance band to a stable object, and then grasp it in one hand. Step back, bending your forward knee.

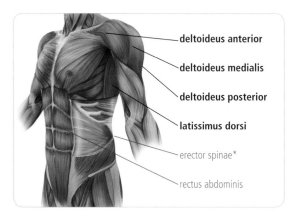

- deltoideus anterior
- deltoideus medialis
- deltoideus posterior
- latissimus dorsi
- erector spinae*
- rectus abdominis

BEST FOR

- deltoideus anterior
- deltoideus medialis
- deltoideus posterior
- latissimus dorsi

ANNOTATION KEY

Black text indicates target muscles
Gray text indicates other working muscles
* indicates deep muscles

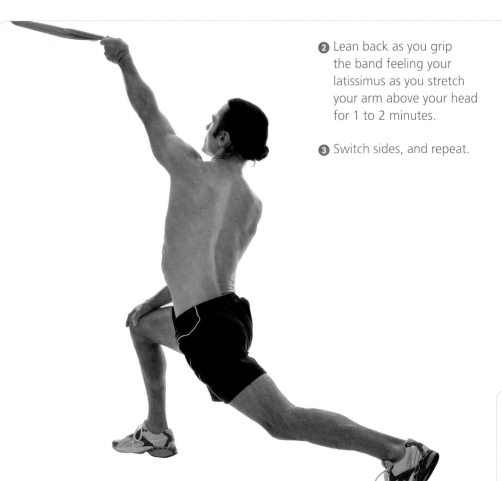

2 Lean back as you grip the band feeling your latissimus as you stretch your arm above your head for 1 to 2 minutes.

3 Switch sides, and repeat.

AVOID
- Pulling too hard, which may place too much stress on your rotator cuff.

TARGETS
- Shoulders
- Back

LEVEL
- Beginner

BENEFITS
- Increases shoulder mobility

NOT ADVISABLE IF YOU HAVE . . .
- Rotator cuff or shoulder injury

DO IT RIGHT
- Use slow and gentle movements.
- Be sure to lean back and feel the stretch in your back and shoulder muscles.

THREAD THE NEEDLE

① Begin on all fours with your back flat and your breathing relaxed.

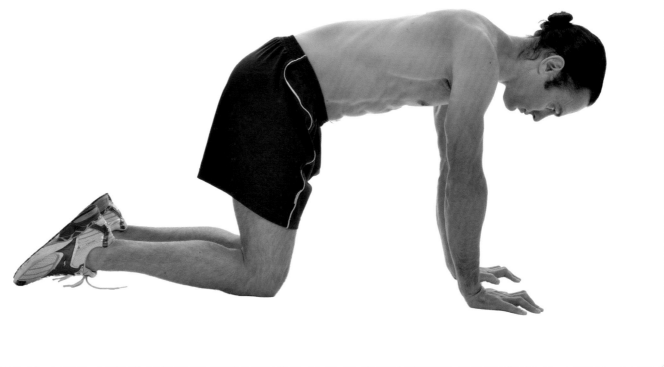

TARGETS
• Back
• Abdominals

LEVEL
• Beginner

BENEFITS
• Improves back mobility

NOT ADVISABLE IF YOU HAVE . . .
• Knee issues
• Rotator cuff injury

② Reach one arm underneath your chest while rotating through, until your forearm rests on the floor.

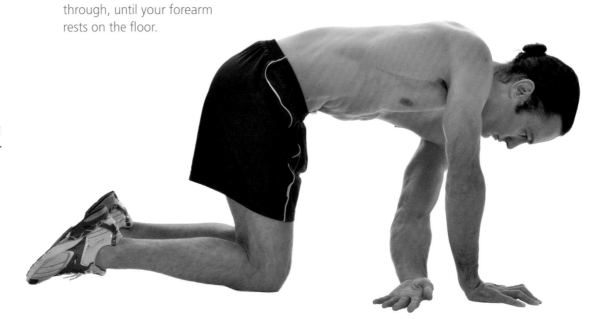

DO IT RIGHT
• Rotate evenly throughout.

③ Hold the stretch for 1 to 2 minutes, and then repeat on the other side.

BEST FOR

• latissimus dorsi
• rectus abdominis
• erector spinae

AVOID
• Speeding through the exercise without completing the full range of motion.

ANNOTATION KEY

Black text indicates target muscles
Gray text indicates other working muscles
* indicates deep muscles

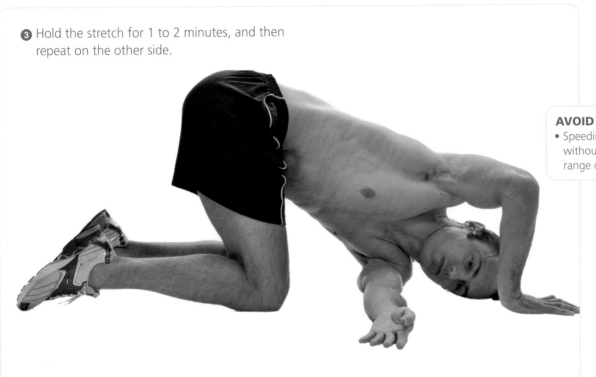

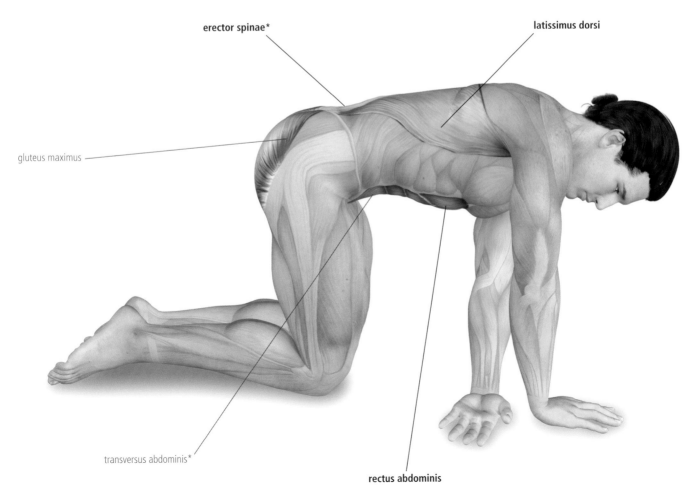

erector spinae*

latissimus dorsi

gluteus maximus

transversus abdominis*

rectus abdominis

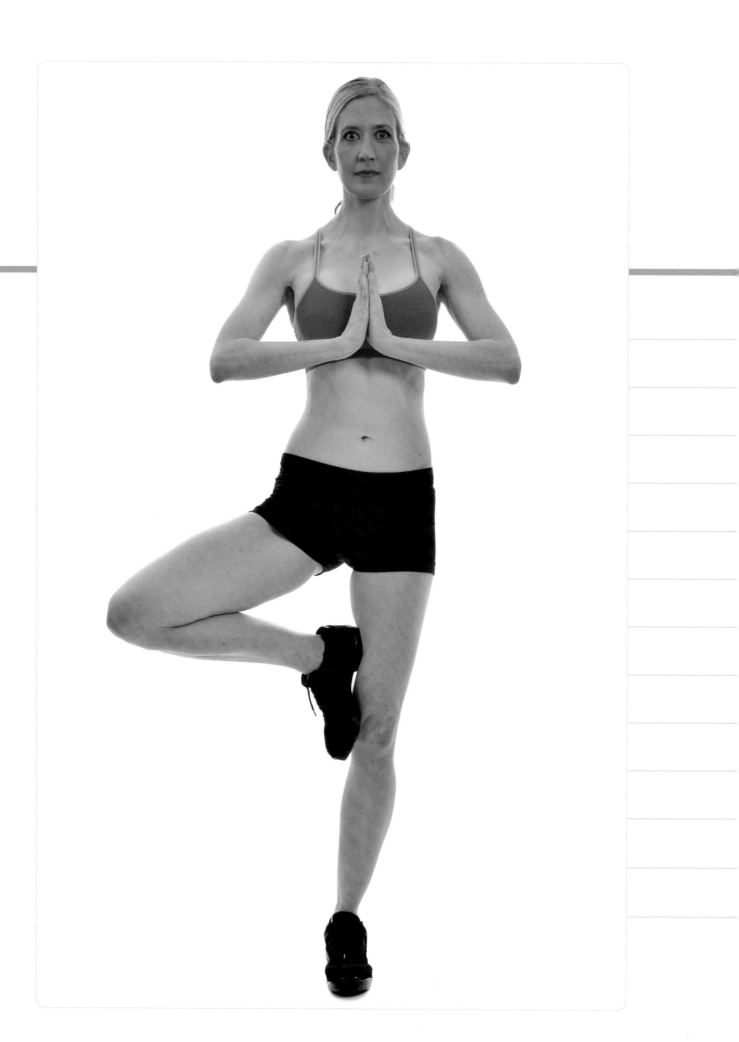

YOGA EXERCISES

Conducted through a series of transitions and poses, for many, yoga is indeed

a very serious and deep way of life. Using mainly one's own body and an

open mind and spirit, the basic goal is enlightenment and unification and the

declaration that the mind, body and spirit are indeed unified as one. Although

yoga is a highly spiritual, emotional and personal journey, it is also a superb

form of exercise that promotes flexibility, balance and strength. It is a perfect

exercise modality for older folk, too, offering low-impact exercises that use

both breathing and the body to bring clarity to the mind.

CHILD'S POSE

❶ Begin on your hands and knees with your knees spaced apart and your toes together.

DO IT RIGHT
- Release any tension from your facial and jaw muscles.
- Face the floor throughout the stretch.

AVOID
- Spacing your knees too far apart.

TARGETS
- Back
- Shoulders

LEVEL
- Beginner

BENEFITS
- Helps keep back muscles flexible

NOT ADVISABLE IF YOU HAVE . . .
- Lower-back issues

❷ Sit your hips back onto your heels while leaning your torso forward and placing your stomach on your thighs.

❸ Place your arms by your sides with the palms facing upward while gently resting your forehead on the floor. Hold for 10 to 30 seconds.

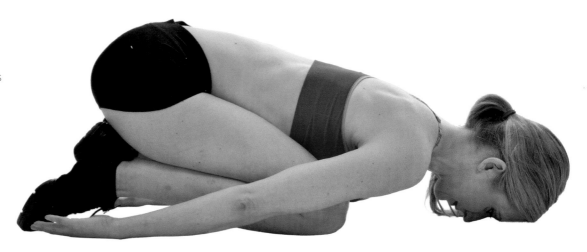

MODIFICATION

Easier: Kneel on all fours, and then sit your hips back onto your heels while leaning your torso forward and placing your stomach on your thighs. Extend your arms straight in front of you.

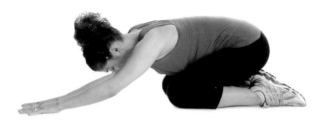

BEST FOR

- **erector spinae**
- **latissimus dorsi**
- **deltoideus posterior**

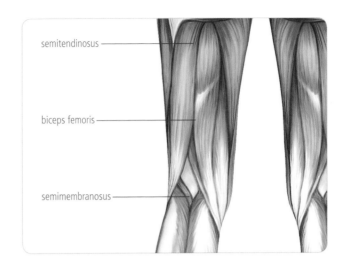

semitendinosus

biceps femoris

semimembranosus

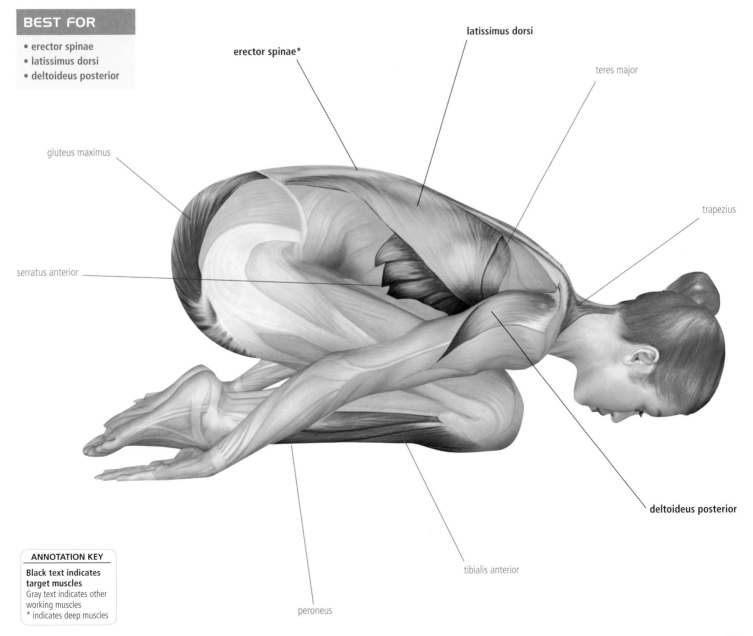

erector spinae*

latissimus dorsi

teres major

gluteus maximus

trapezius

serratus anterior

deltoideus posterior

tibialis anterior

peroneus

ANNOTATION KEY

Black text indicates target muscles
Gray text indicates other working muscles
* indicates deep muscles

DOWNWARD-FACING DOG

① Begin on your hands and knees, with your hands aligned under your shoulders and your knees under your hips.

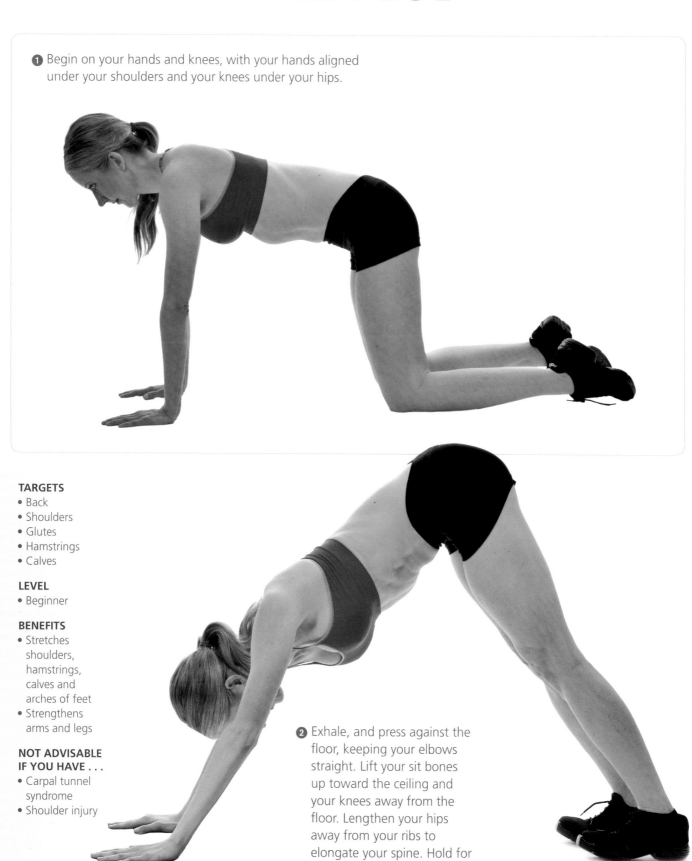

TARGETS
• Back
• Shoulders
• Glutes
• Hamstrings
• Calves

LEVEL
• Beginner

BENEFITS
• Stretches shoulders, hamstrings, calves and arches of feet
• Strengthens arms and legs

NOT ADVISABLE IF YOU HAVE . . .
• Carpal tunnel syndrome
• Shoulder injury

② Exhale, and press against the floor, keeping your elbows straight. Lift your sit bones up toward the ceiling and your knees away from the floor. Lengthen your hips away from your ribs to elongate your spine. Hold for 30 seconds to 2 minutes.

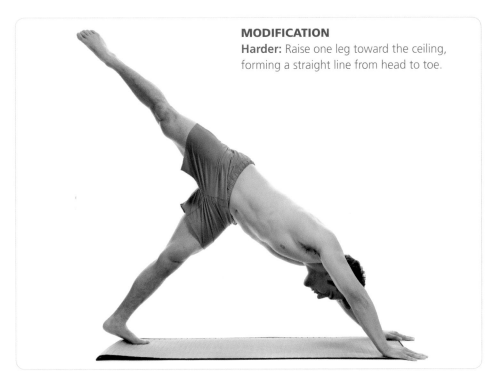

MODIFICATION

Harder: Raise one leg toward the ceiling, forming a straight line from head to toe.

BEST FOR

- triceps brachii
- deltoideus posterior
- latissimus dorsi
- semitendinosus
- biceps femoris
- semimembranosus

AVOID

- Sinking your shoulders into your armpits, creating an arch in your back.
- Rounding your spine

DO IT RIGHT

- Contract your thigh muscles to further lengthen your spine and keep pressure off your shoulders.
- Press your heels into the floor.

ANNOTATION KEY

Black text indicates target muscles
Gray text indicates other working muscles
* indicates deep muscles

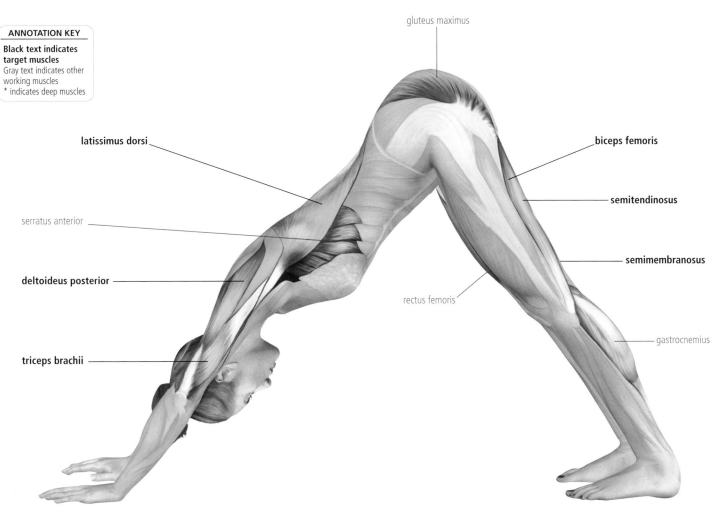

gluteus maximus

latissimus dorsi

biceps femoris

semitendinosus

serratus anterior

deltoideus posterior

semimembranosus

rectus femoris

triceps brachii

gastrocnemius

HIGH LUNGE

❶ Stand with your feet together and your arms hanging at your sides.

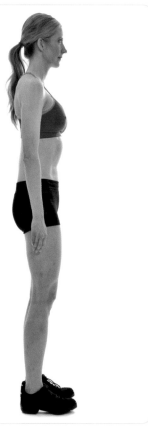

❷ Exhale, and carefully step back with your right leg, keeping it in line with your hips as you step back. The ball of your left foot should be in contact with the floor as you do the motion.

❸ Slowly slide your right foot farther back while bending your left knee, stacking it directly above your ankle.

❹ Position your palms or fingers on the floor on either side of your left leg, and slowly press your palms or fingers against the floor to enhance the placement of your upper body and your head.

❺ Lift your head and gaze straight forward while leaning your upper body forward and carefully rolling your shoulders down and backward.

❻ Press the ball of your right foot gradually into the floor, contract your thigh muscles, and press up to keep your left leg straight.

❼ Hold for 5 to 10 seconds. Slowly return to the starting position, and then repeat on the other side.

TARGETS
- Quadriceps
- Hamstrings
- Calf muscles

LEVEL
- Beginner

BENEFITS
- Strengthens legs and arms
- Stretches groins

NOT ADVISABLE IF YOU HAVE . . .
- Arm injury
- Shoulder injury
- Hip injury

DO IT RIGHT
- Keep your thighs taut as you stretch.

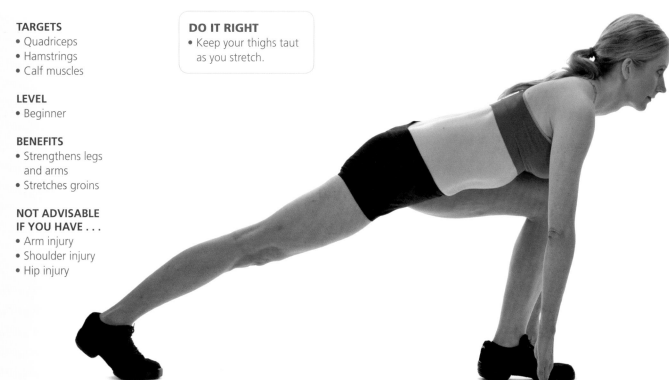

AVOID
• Dropping your back knee to the floor.
• Hyperextending your knee past your ankle.

BEST FOR
• gastrocnemius
• soleus
• tibialis posterior
• rectus femoris
• vastus lateralis
• vastus intermedius
• vastus medialis
• gluteus maximus

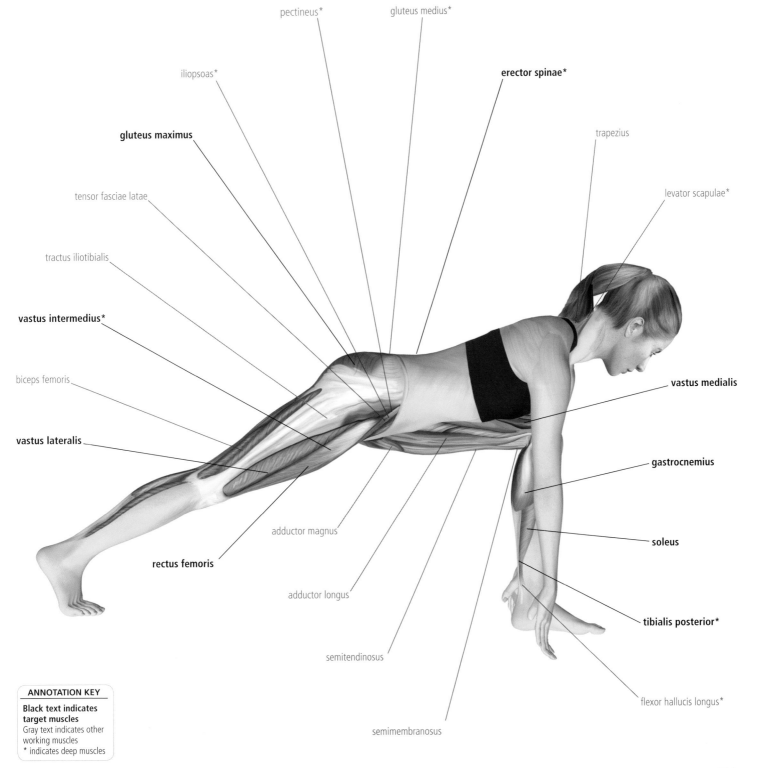

pectineus*

gluteus medius*

iliopsoas*

erector spinae*

gluteus maximus

trapezius

tensor fasciae latae

levator scapulae*

tractus iliotibialis

vastus intermedius*

vastus medialis

biceps femoris

vastus lateralis

gastrocnemius

adductor magnus

rectus femoris

soleus

adductor longus

tibialis posterior*

semitendinosus

flexor hallucis longus*

semimembranosus

ANNOTATION KEY
Black text indicates target muscles
Gray text indicates other working muscles
* indicates deep muscles

UPWARD SALUTE

❶ Stand tall with your arms at your sides.

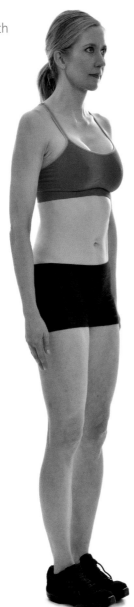

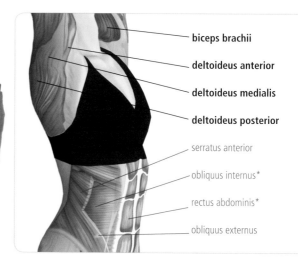

- biceps brachii
- deltoideus anterior
- deltoideus medialis
- deltoideus posterior
- serratus anterior
- obliquus internus*
- rectus abdominis*
- obliquus externus

ANNOTATION KEY

Black text indicates target muscles
Gray text indicates other working muscles
* indicates deep muscles

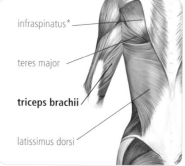

- infraspinatus*
- teres major
- **triceps brachii**
- latissimus dorsi

TARGETS
- Shoulders
- Abdominals

LEVEL
- Beginner

BENEFITS
- Alleviates backache
- Stretches abdominals
- Stretches shoulders and armpits
- Opens up entire body

NOT ADVISABLE IF YOU HAVE . . .
- Shoulder injury
- Neck injury

❷ Inhale, and raise your arms out to your sides, elongating your torso and continuing to raise your arms until they are directly above your head.

❸ Lengthen your arms with your palms facing each other, and hold for 10 to 30 seconds.

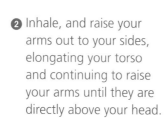

DO IT RIGHT
- Keep your shoulders aligned directly over your hips and your hips over your heels.
- Keep back ribs broad.
- Broaden the top of your shoulder blades.
- Move your armpits down while lifting the arms upward.

AVOID
- Jutting your rib cage out of your chest.
- Shrugging your shoulders up to your ears.

BEST FOR

- triceps brachii
- biceps brachii
- deltoideus anterior
- deltoideus medialis
- deltoideus posterior

TREE POSE

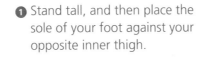

1. Stand tall, and then place the sole of your foot against your opposite inner thigh.

2. Keep your abdominals braced and bring your hands together in a prayer position. Hold the pose for 10 to 30 seconds, and then repeat on the other leg.

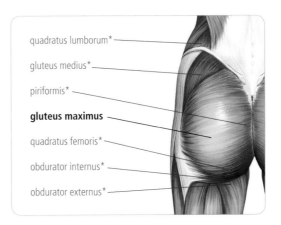

quadratus lumborum*
gluteus medius*
piriformis*
gluteus maximus
quadratus femoris*
obdurator internus*
obdurator externus*

ANNOTATION KEY

Black text indicates target muscles
Gray text indicates other working muscles
* indicates deep muscles

BEST FOR

- gastrocnemius
- soleus
- tibialis anterior
- rectus femoris
- vastus lateralis
- vastus intermedius
- vastus medialis
- gluteus maximus
- iliopsoas

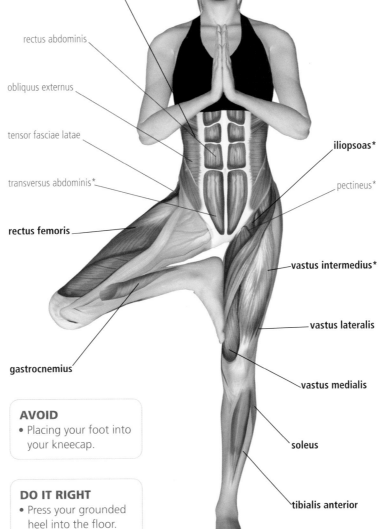

obliquus internus*
rectus abdominis
obliquus externus
tensor fasciae latae
transversus abdominis*
rectus femoris
gastrocnemius

iliopsoas*
pectineus*
vastus intermedius*
vastus lateralis
vastus medialis
soleus
tibialis anterior

TARGETS
- Legs
- Glutes

LEVEL
- Beginner

BENEFITS
- Strengthens thighs, calves, ankles and spine
- Stretches groin, inner thighs, chest and shoulders
- Improves sense of balance
- Relieves sciatica
- Reduces flat feet

NOT ADVISABLE IF YOU HAVE . . .
- High or low blood pressure

MODIFICATION
Similar level of difficulty:
Raise your arms upward with your palms facing each other.

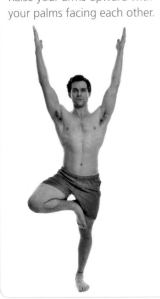

AVOID
- Placing your foot into your kneecap.

DO IT RIGHT
- Press your grounded heel into the floor.

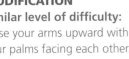

PLANK POSE

1 Begin on the floor with your hands flat and your legs elongated and balanced on your toes with your heels pressing outward. Your spine should be in one long line and your arms parallel to each other.

2 Hold this position for 10 to 30 seconds as you lift your sternum and lengthen your tailbone.

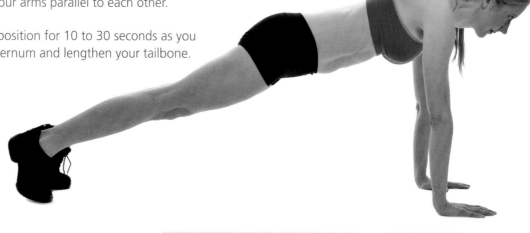

BEST FOR

- triceps brachii
- deltoideus anterior
- pectoralis major
- pectoralis minor
- erector spinae
- gluteus maximus
- biceps femoris
- semitendinosus
- semimembranosus
- gastrocnemius
- trapezius
- rectus abdominis

DO IT RIGHT
- Keep your body one long length.
- Spread your fingers wide, and ground down through each knuckle.
- Use your breath to get you through holding the pose.

AVOID
- Rounding your back.
- Squeeze your glutes.

ANNOTATION KEY
Black text indicates target muscles
Gray text indicates other working muscles
* indicates deep muscles

TARGETS
- Chest
- Upper arms
- Core

LEVEL
- Beginner

BENEFITS
- Strengthens arms, chest and core stabilizers

NOT ADVISABLE IF YOU HAVE . . .
- Shoulder issues
- Wrist pain
- Lower-back pain

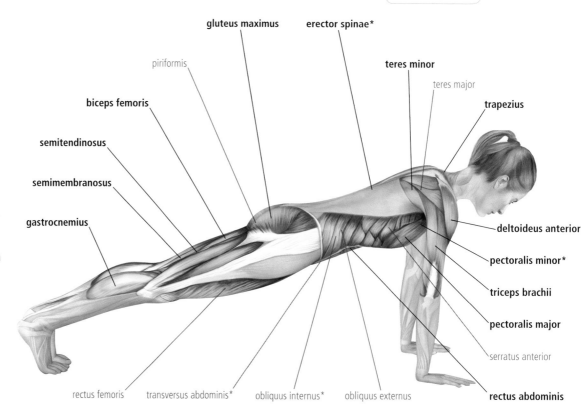

gluteus maximus

erector spinae*

teres minor

teres major

trapezius

piriformis

biceps femoris

semitendinosus

semimembranosus

deltoideus anterior

gastrocnemius

pectoralis minor*

triceps brachii

pectoralis major

serratus anterior

rectus abdominis

rectus femoris   transversus abdominis*   obliquus internus*   obliquus externus

CHATURANGA

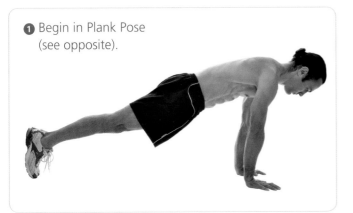

❶ Begin in Plank Pose (see opposite).

AVOID
- Rounding your back.
- Dropping your hips lower than your shoulders.

DO IT RIGHT
- Keep your body one long length.
- Spread your fingers wide, and ground down through each knuckle.
- Use your breath to get you through holding the pose.

BEST FOR
- triceps brachii
- deltoideus posterior
- pectoralis major
- obliquus externus
- obliquus internus
- serratus anterior

ANNOTATION KEY

Black text indicates target muscles
Gray text indicates other working muscles
* indicates deep muscles

---

❷ Exhale as you lower yourself to the floor, pushing your palms into the ground until your elbows are in line with your shoulders. Keep your body in one straight line and your spine long as you hold for 10 to 30 seconds.

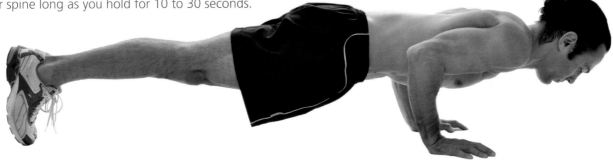

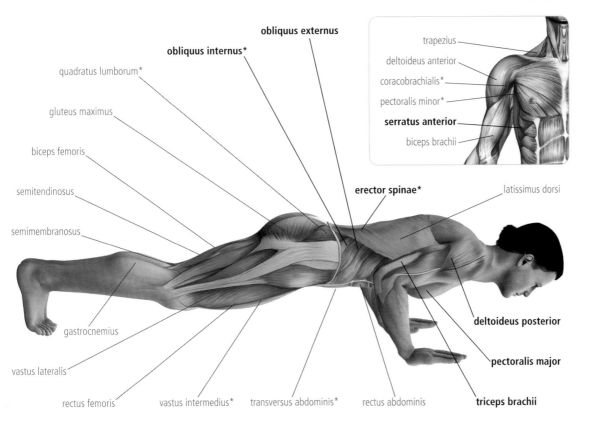

obliquus externus

obliquus internus*

quadratus lumborum*

gluteus maximus

biceps femoris

semitendinosus

semimembranosus

gastrocnemius

vastus lateralis

rectus femoris

vastus intermedius*

transversus abdominis*

rectus abdominis

erector spinae*

latissimus dorsi

trapezius

deltoideus anterior

coracobrachialis*

pectoralis minor*

serratus anterior

biceps brachii

deltoideus posterior

pectoralis major

triceps brachii

TARGETS
- Chest
- Upper arms

LEVEL
- Intermediate

BENEFITS
- Strengthens the core stabilizers, shoulders, back, buttocks and pectoral muscles

NOT ADVISABLE IF YOU HAVE . . .
- Shoulder issues
- Wrist pain
- Lower-back pain

UPWARD-FACING DOG

1 Begin in Chaturanga (see page 89), supporting your weight evenly between your hands and feet

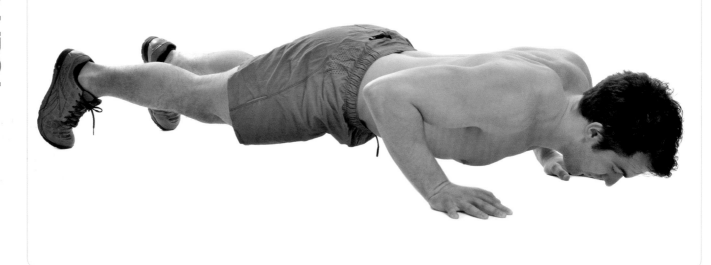

TARGETS
- Back
- Abdominals

LEVEL
- Beginner

BENEFITS
- Stretches chest, shoulders, thighs and abdomen
- Strengthens wrists, arms and spine
- Improves posture

NOT ADVISABLE IF YOU HAVE . . .
- Back injury
- Wrist injury or carpal tunnel syndrome

2 Raise your head as you flip the tops of your feet to the floor and straighten your arms with your shoulders above your wrists.

DO IT RIGHT
- Elongate your legs and arms to create full extension.
- Make sure that your wrists are positioned directly below your shoulders so that you don't exert too much pressure on your lower back.

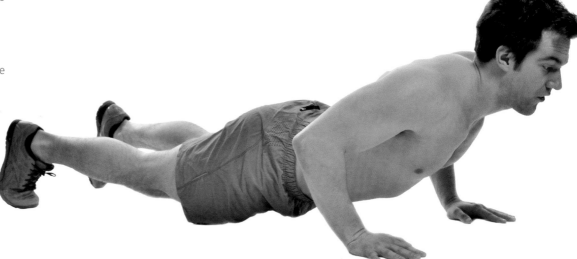

3 Keeping your knees and thighs off the floor, lift your hips and look upward. Hold this position for 10 to 15 seconds.

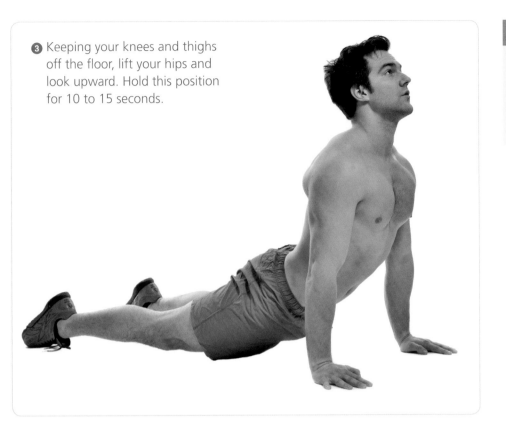

BEST FOR

- erector spinae
- rhomboideus
- teres major
- teres minor
- trapezius
- latissimus dorsi
- quadratus lumborum
- gluteus maximus
- pectoralis major
- serratus anterior
- rectus abdominis
- triceps brachii

AVOID
- Lifting your shoulders up toward your ears.
- Hyperextending your elbows.
- Jutting your rib cage out of your chest.
- Dropping your thighs or knees to the floor.

ANNOTATION KEY
Black text indicates target muscles
Gray text indicates other working muscles
* indicates deep muscles

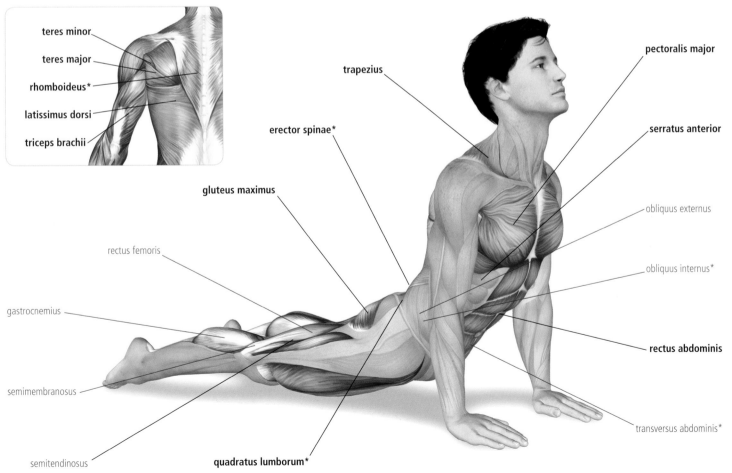

teres minor

teres major

rhomboideus*

latissimus dorsi

triceps brachii

trapezius

erector spinae*

gluteus maximus

rectus femoris

gastrocnemius

semimembranosus

semitendinosus

quadratus lumborum*

pectoralis major

serratus anterior

obliquus externus

obliquus internus*

rectus abdominis

transversus abdominis*

SIDE-ANGLE POSE

1 Begin in an upright position with your feet spread apart and one foot turned outward while the other faces forward.

2 Extend your arms directly out to your sides with your palms facing downward. Bend your forward knee until it's positioned above your ankle

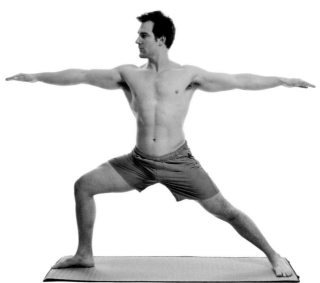

DO IT RIGHT
- Keep your leading knee tight and aligned with the center of your leading foot, shin and thigh.
- Bend from your hips, not your waist.
- If you feel unsteady, brace your back heel against a wall.

3 Bend your torso toward your bent knee, reaching your fingers to the floor as you raise your opposite arm straight toward the ceiling. Take 5 slow breaths, then return to the standing position and switch sides.

TARGETS
- Core
- Hips

LEVEL
- Beginner

BENEFITS
- Strengthens core
- Opens hips
- Stretches thighs, knees, ankles, hips, groin, hamstrings, calves, shoulders, chest and spine
- Relieves the symptoms of menopause

NOT ADVISABLE IF YOU HAVE . . .
- High or low blood pressure
- Neck issues

AVOID
- Twisting your hips.
- Leaning forward—keep your hips and shoulders aligned.

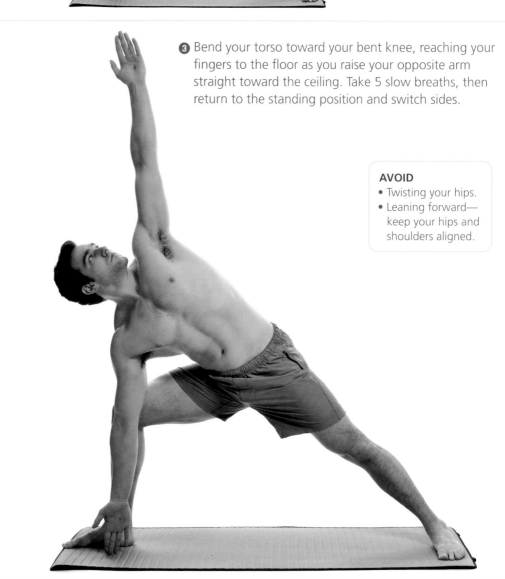

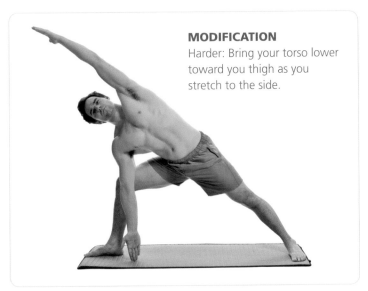

MODIFICATION

Harder: Bring your torso lower toward you thigh as you stretch to the side.

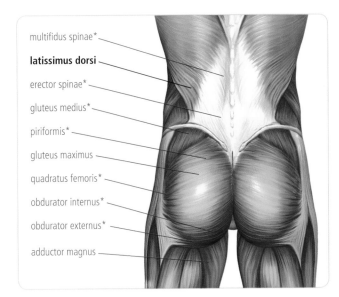

multifidus spinae*

latissimus dorsi

erector spinae*

gluteus medius*

piriformis*

gluteus maximus

quadratus femoris*

obdurator internus*

obdurator externus*

adductor magnus

BEST FOR

• adductor longus
• sartorius
• latissimus dorsi
• serratus anterior
• rectus abdominis
• obliquus externus
• obliquus internus

ANNOTATION KEY

Black text indicates target muscles
Gray text indicates other working muscles
* indicates deep muscles

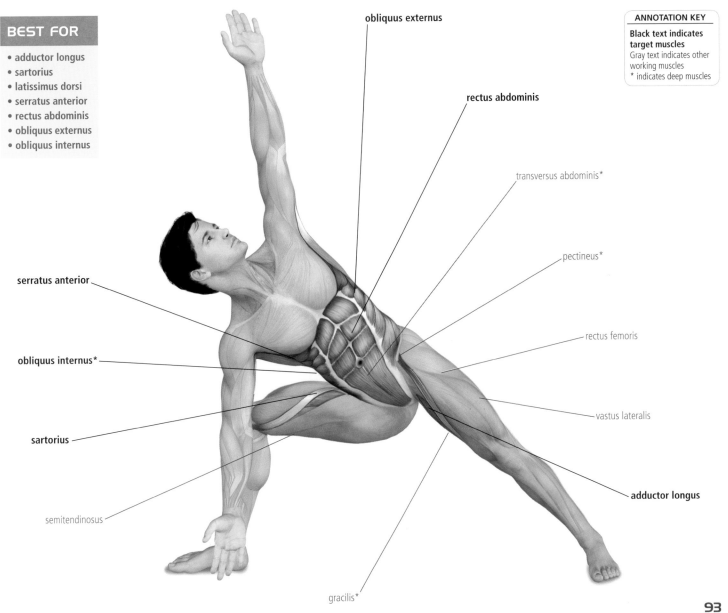

obliquus externus

rectus abdominis

transversus abdominis*

pectineus*

rectus femoris

vastus lateralis

serratus anterior

obliquus internus*

sartorius

semitendinosus

adductor longus

gracilis*

CHAIR POSE

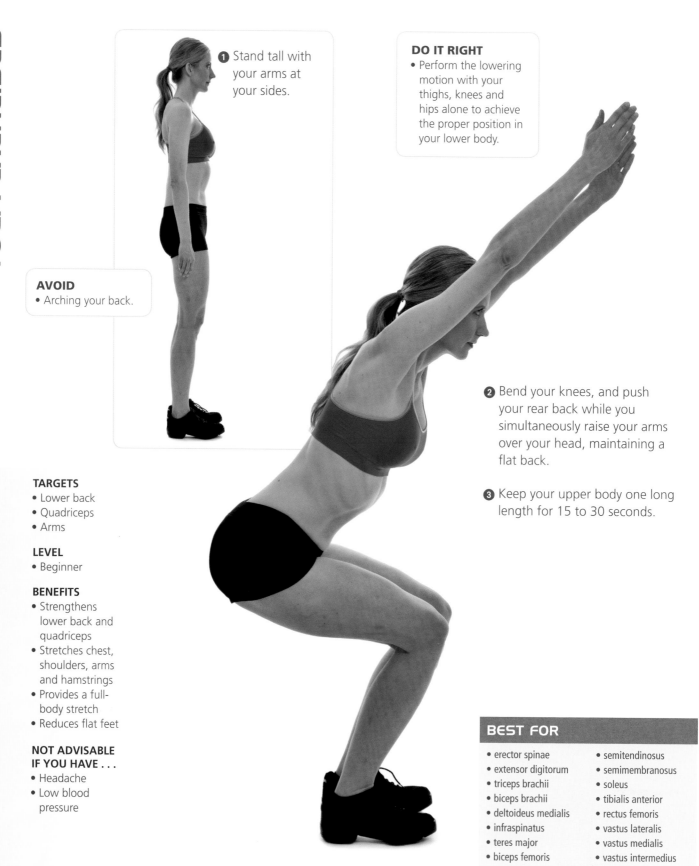

❶ Stand tall with your arms at your sides.

DO IT RIGHT
• Perform the lowering motion with your thighs, knees and hips alone to achieve the proper position in your lower body.

AVOID
• Arching your back.

❷ Bend your knees, and push your rear back while you simultaneously raise your arms over your head, maintaining a flat back.

❸ Keep your upper body one long length for 15 to 30 seconds.

TARGETS
• Lower back
• Quadriceps
• Arms

LEVEL
• Beginner

BENEFITS
• Strengthens lower back and quadriceps
• Stretches chest, shoulders, arms and hamstrings
• Provides a full-body stretch
• Reduces flat feet

NOT ADVISABLE IF YOU HAVE . . .
• Headache
• Low blood pressure

BEST FOR

• erector spinae	• semitendinosus
• extensor digitorum	• semimembranosus
• triceps brachii	• soleus
• biceps brachii	• tibialis anterior
• deltoideus medialis	• rectus femoris
• infraspinatus	• vastus lateralis
• teres major	• vastus medialis
• biceps femoris	• vastus intermedius

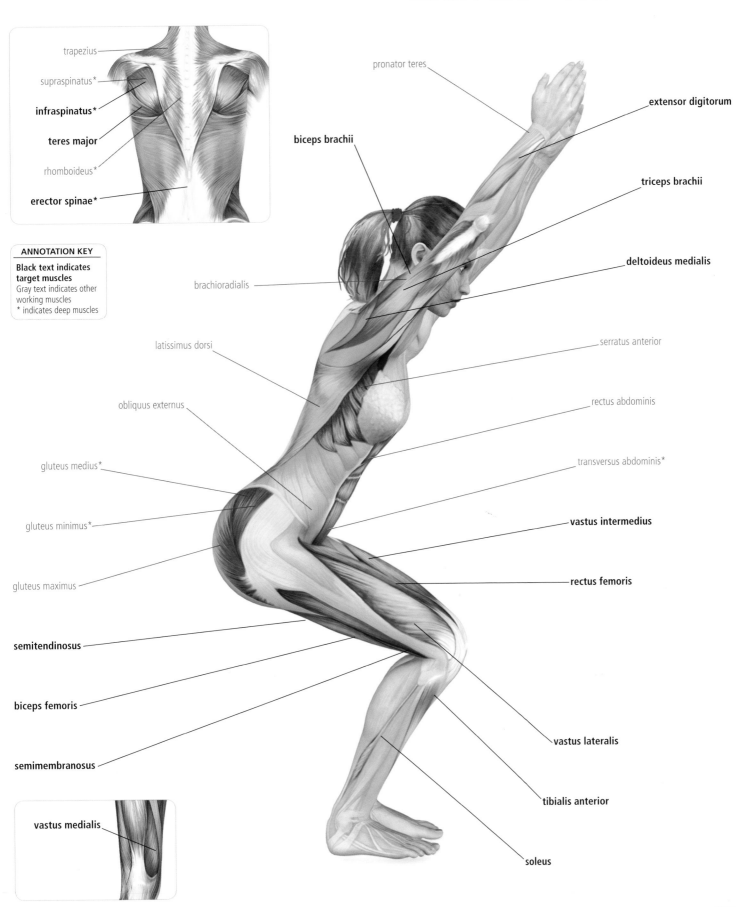

trapezius

supraspinatus*

infraspinatus*

teres major

rhomboideus*

erector spinae*

ANNOTATION KEY
**Black text indicates
target muscles**
Gray text indicates other
working muscles
* indicates deep muscles

pronator teres

extensor digitorum

biceps brachii

triceps brachii

brachioradialis

deltoideus medialis

latissimus dorsi

serratus anterior

obliquus externus

rectus abdominis

gluteus medius*

transversus abdominis*

gluteus minimus*

vastus intermedius

gluteus maximus

rectus femoris

semitendinosus

biceps femoris

vastus lateralis

semimembranosus

tibialis anterior

vastus medialis

soleus

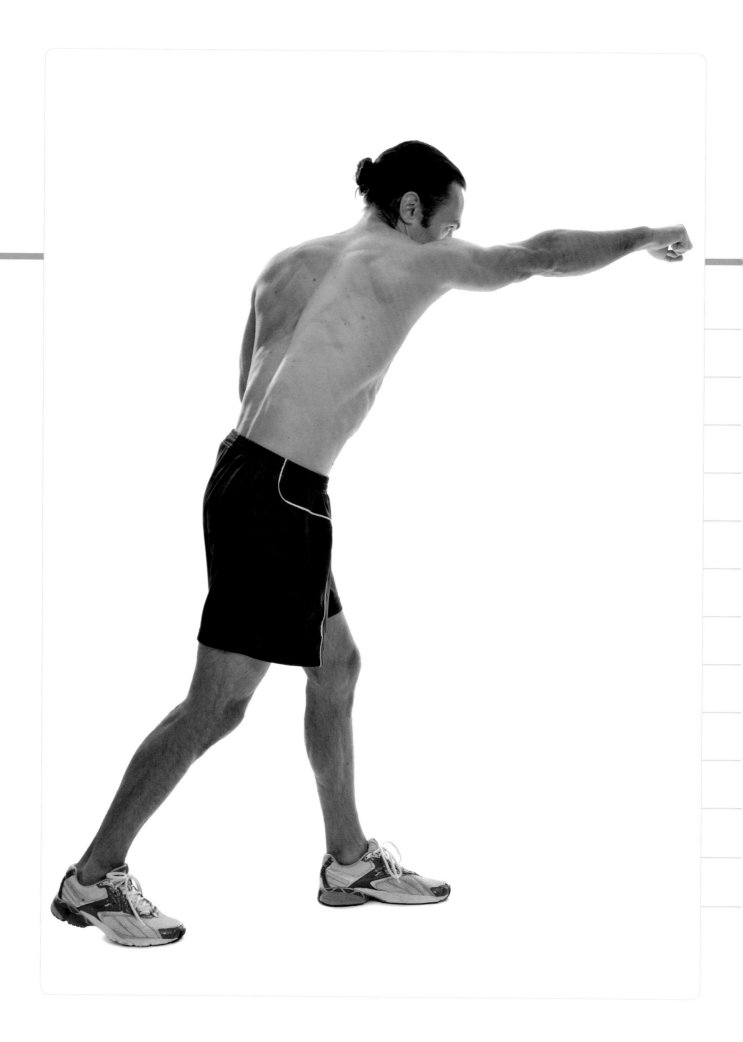

CARDIO EXERCISES

Cardio exercise, also called cardiovascular or cardiorespiratory exercise, is designed to get your heart rate up, which improves oxygen consumption in your body. Cardio is an essential part of the longevity program because it helps build endurance, keeping you fit and active in all parts of your life. It also helps you to lose extra fat or maintain a healthy weight.

The following exercises rely on body weight to supply resistance. If you want to try something different and refuse to pedal one more rep on the stationary bike or walk one more step on the treadmill, this group is your ticket to progress and a new sense of self. You can easily modify them to suit any fitness level, and you can increase the challenge simply by adding more time and going at them longer. Your heart and body will thank you.

HIGH KNEES

1 Stand tall with your hands either on your hips or down by your sides.

2 Raise up one knee as high as you are able, and then return to the starting position.

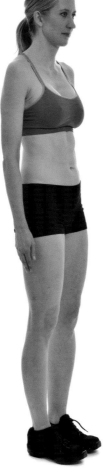
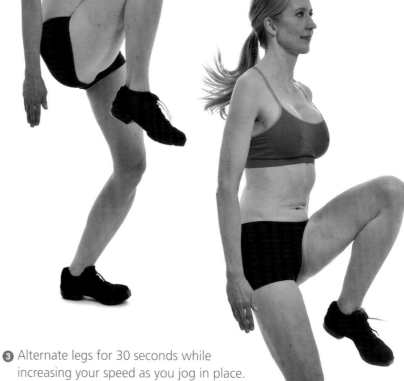

3 Alternate legs for 30 seconds while increasing your speed as you jog in place.

TARGETS
- Glutes
- Quadriceps
- Hamstrings
- Calves

LEVEL
- Beginner

BENEFITS
- Strengthens lower body
- Serves as a warm-up for other exercise
- Builds endurance

NOT ADVISABLE IF YOU HAVE . . .
- Knee issues
- Ankle pain

AVOID
- Pushing solely off your toes.

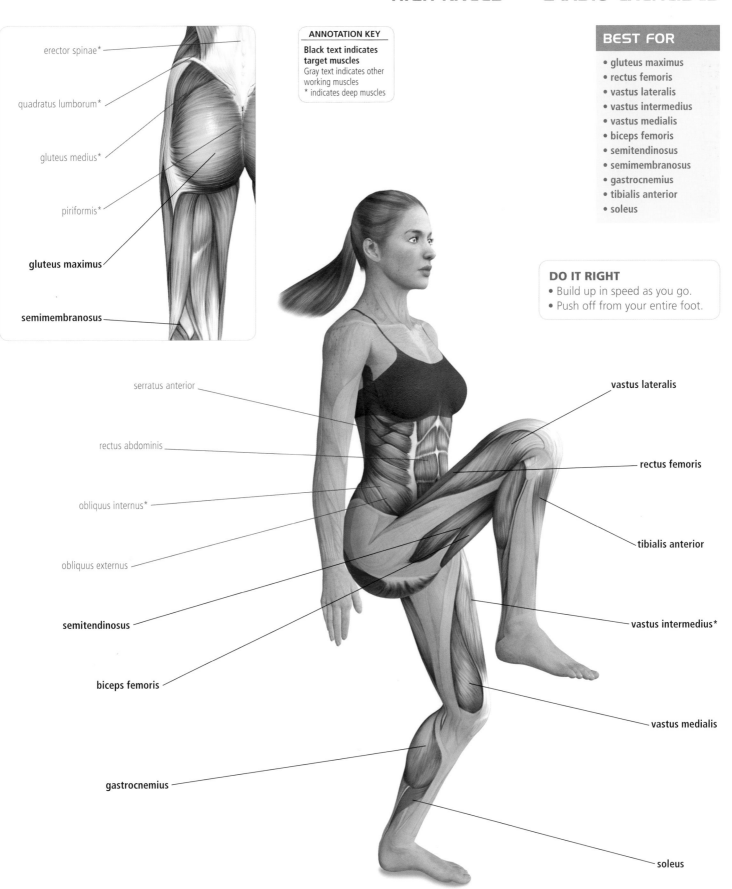

ANNOTATION KEY

Black text indicates target muscles
Gray text indicates other working muscles
* indicates deep muscles

erector spinae*

quadratus lumborum*

gluteus medius*

piriformis*

gluteus maximus

semimembranosus

BEST FOR

- gluteus maximus
- rectus femoris
- vastus lateralis
- vastus intermedius
- vastus medialis
- biceps femoris
- semitendinosus
- semimembranosus
- gastrocnemius
- tibialis anterior
- soleus

DO IT RIGHT
- Build up in speed as you go.
- Push off from your entire foot.

serratus anterior

rectus abdominis

obliquus internus*

obliquus externus

semitendinosus

biceps femoris

gastrocnemius

vastus lateralis

rectus femoris

tibialis anterior

vastus intermedius*

vastus medialis

soleus

INCHWORM

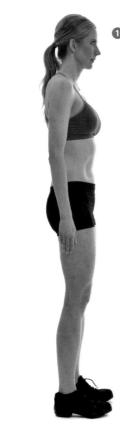

1 Begin in a standing position.

2 Bend forward, touching your fingertips to the floor.

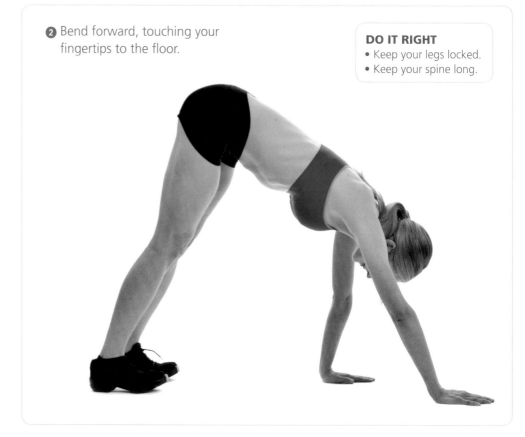

DO IT RIGHT
- Keep your legs locked.
- Keep your spine long.

3 Start walking your hands forward.

AVOID
- Excessive momentum.
- Falling into your shoulders on the push-up portion of the exercise.

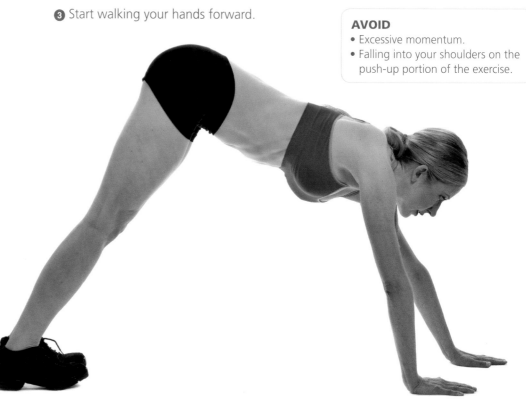

TARGETS
- Back
- Shoulders
- Abdominals
- Hamstrings
- Calves

LEVEL
- Beginner

BENEFITS
- Builds endurance
- Increases coordination

NOT ADVISABLE IF YOU HAVE . . .
- Arm injury
- Shoulder injury
- Hip injury
- High or low blood pressure

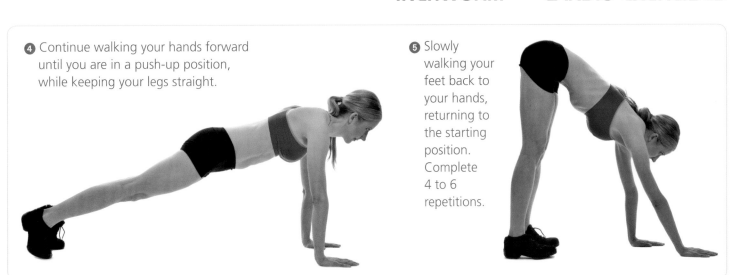

④ Continue walking your hands forward until you are in a push-up position, while keeping your legs straight.

⑤ Slowly walking your feet back to your hands, returning to the starting position. Complete 4 to 6 repetitions.

BEST FOR

- deltoideus anterior
- deltoideus medialis
- deltoideus posterior
- latissimus dorsi
- rectus abdominis
- erector spinae
- gluteus maximus
- biceps femoris
- semitendinosus
- semimembranosus
- gastrocnemius
- tibialis anterior
- soleus

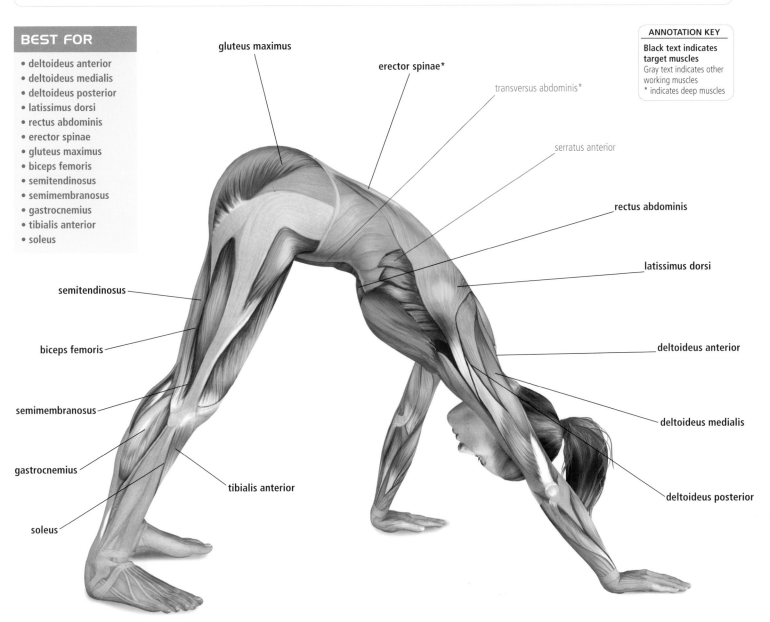

gluteus maximus

erector spinae*

transversus abdominis*

serratus anterior

rectus abdominis

latissimus dorsi

deltoideus anterior

deltoideus medialis

deltoideus posterior

semitendinosus

biceps femoris

semimembranosus

gastrocnemius

tibialis anterior

soleus

BUTT KICK

❶ Begin in a standing position, and then jog in place.

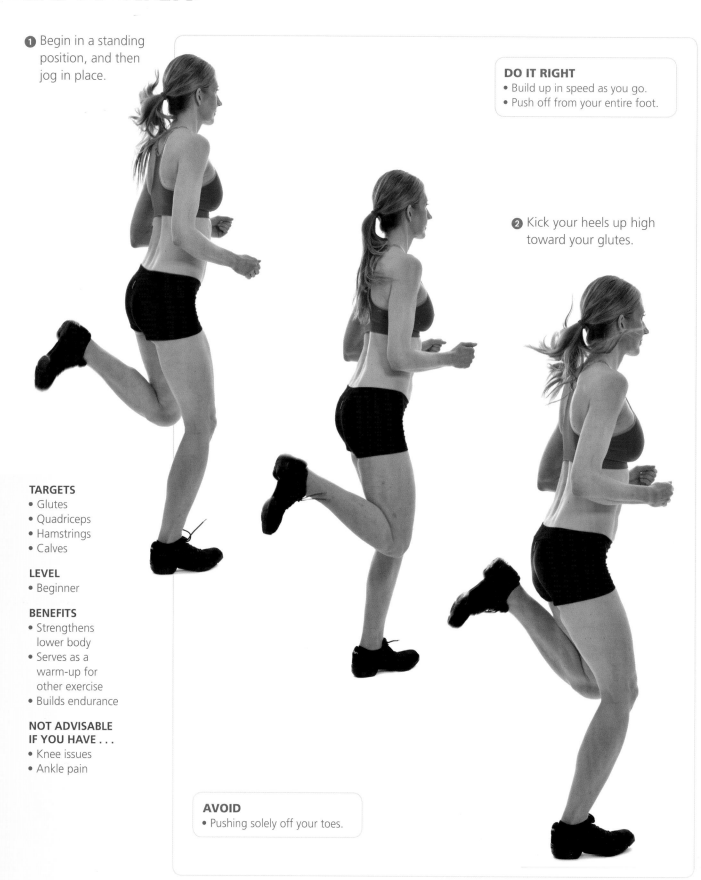

DO IT RIGHT
- Build up in speed as you go.
- Push off from your entire foot.

❷ Kick your heels up high toward your glutes.

TARGETS
- Glutes
- Quadriceps
- Hamstrings
- Calves

LEVEL
- Beginner

BENEFITS
- Strengthens lower body
- Serves as a warm-up for other exercise
- Builds endurance

NOT ADVISABLE IF YOU HAVE . . .
- Knee issues
- Ankle pain

AVOID
- Pushing solely off your toes.

3 Continue jogging in place, lifting your heels high, for up to a minute while increasing your speed as you go.

ANNOTATION KEY

Black text indicates target muscles
Gray text indicates other working muscles
* indicates deep muscles

BEST FOR

- gluteus maximus
- rectus femoris
- vastus lateralis
- vastus intermedius
- vastus medialis
- biceps femoris
- semitendinosus
- semimembranosus
- gastrocnemius
- tibialis anterior
- soleus

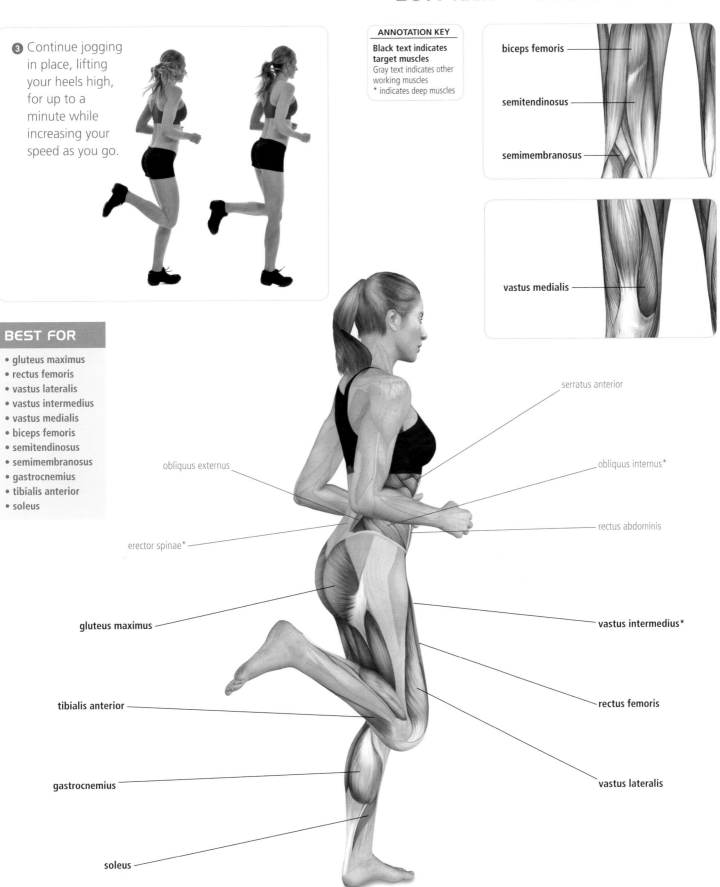

biceps femoris

semitendinosus

semimembranosus

vastus medialis

serratus anterior

obliquus externus

obliquus internus*

rectus abdominis

erector spinae*

gluteus maximus

vastus intermedius*

tibialis anterior

rectus femoris

gastrocnemius

vastus lateralis

soleus

DIVER'S PUSH-UP

① Begin in the Downward-Facing Dog position (see page 82).

AVOID
- Bending your legs.
- Letting your thighs or knees rest on the floor.

DO IT RIGHT
- Position your arms firmly on the floor, securely grounding your fingers.
- Move with control.

② With a controlled movement, swoop your hips toward the floor while simultaneously raising your chest.

TARGETS
- Shoulders
- Hamstrings
- Back
- Abdominals

LEVEL
- Beginner

BENEFITS
- Stretches chest, shoulders, thighs and abdomen
- Strengthens legs, wrists, arms and spine
- Improves posture

NOT ADVISABLE IF YOU HAVE . . .
- Back injury
- Wrist injury or carpal tunnel syndrome

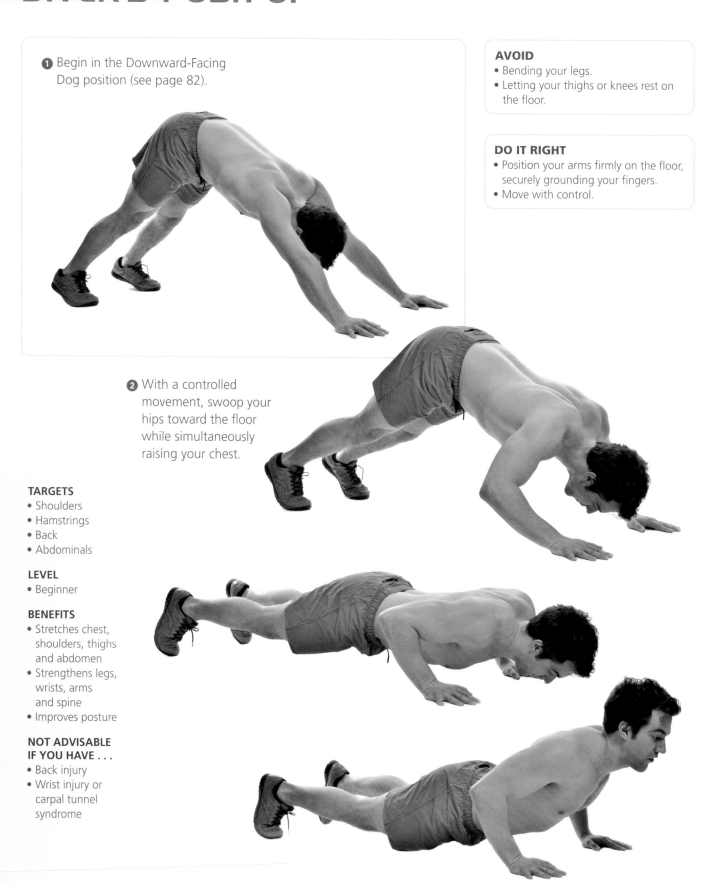

3 Continue rising upward until you're looking toward the ceiling and your back is arched.

4 Swoop back down, and the repeat the entire sequence for 10 to 15 repetitions.

BEST FOR

- triceps brachii
- deltoideus posterior
- latissimus dorsi
- semitendinosus
- biceps femoris
- semimembranosus

ANNOTATION KEY

Black text indicates target muscles
Gray text indicates other working muscles
* indicates deep muscles

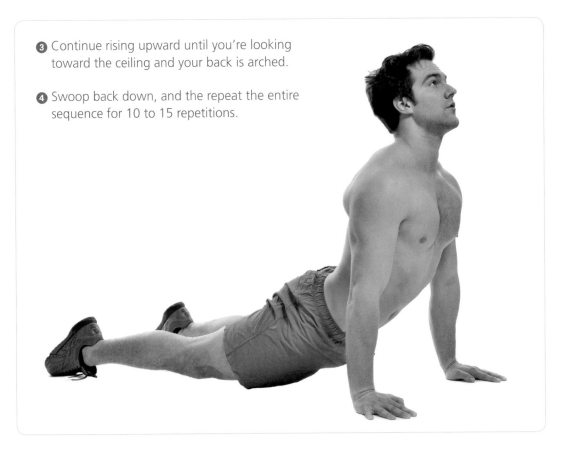

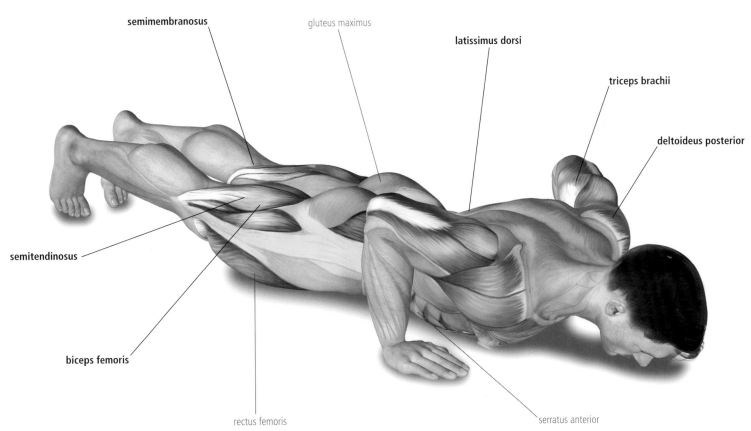

semimembranosus

gluteus maximus

latissimus dorsi

triceps brachii

deltoideus posterior

semitendinosus

biceps femoris

rectus femoris

serratus anterior

STEP-UP

❶ Begin in a standing position behind a flat bench or elevated platform, and place your right foot on it.

❷ Step up onto the bench until your left leg is straight, using your right hamstring and glute to complete the movement. Lower your left leg, and repeat for 10 to 12 repetitions.

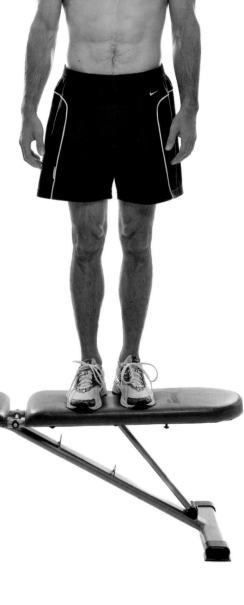

TARGETS
• Quadriceps
• Hamstrings
• Glutes

LEVEL
• Beginner

BENEFITS
• Strengthens thighs, glutes and hamstrings
• Builds endurance

NOT ADVISABLE IF YOU HAVE . . .
• Knee issues

❸ Switch starting position with your left leg on the bench, and repeat on the other side.

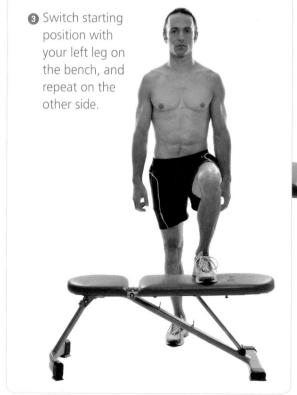

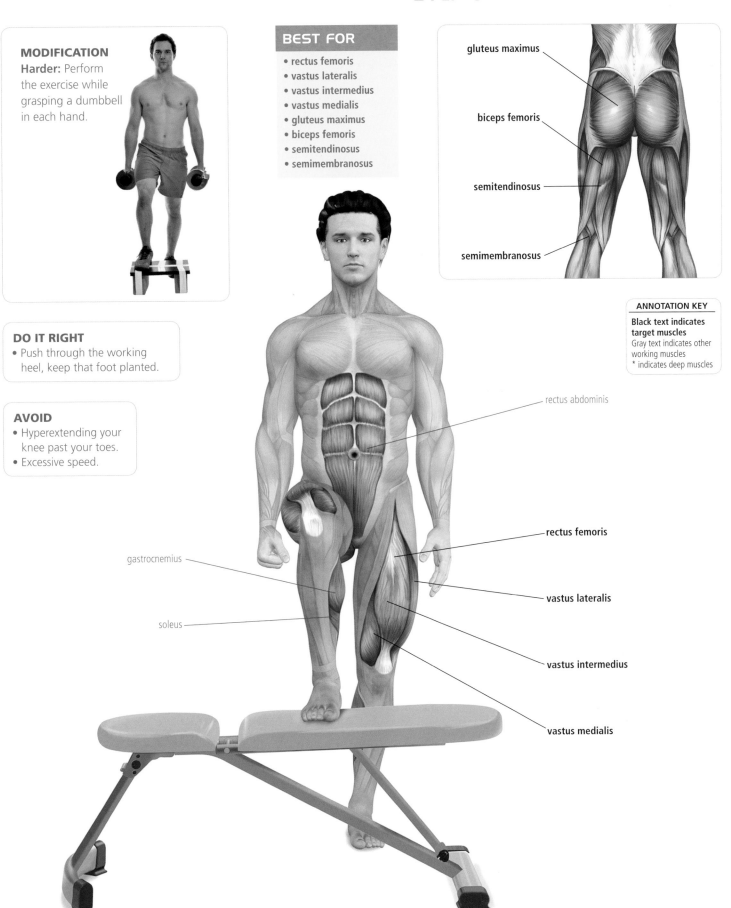

MODIFICATION
Harder: Perform the exercise while grasping a dumbbell in each hand.

BEST FOR
- rectus femoris
- vastus lateralis
- vastus intermedius
- vastus medialis
- gluteus maximus
- biceps femoris
- semitendinosus
- semimembranosus

gluteus maximus

biceps femoris

semitendinosus

semimembranosus

ANNOTATION KEY

Black text indicates target muscles
Gray text indicates other working muscles
* indicates deep muscles

DO IT RIGHT
- Push through the working heel, keep that foot planted.

AVOID
- Hyperextending your knee past your toes.
- Excessive speed.

rectus abdominis

rectus femoris

vastus lateralis

gastrocnemius

vastus intermedius

soleus

vastus medialis

SKATER'S LUNGE

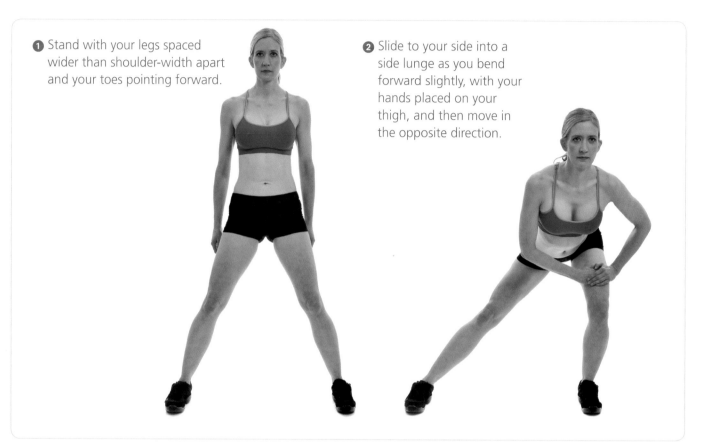

1 Stand with your legs spaced wider than shoulder-width apart and your toes pointing forward.

2 Slide to your side into a side lunge as you bend forward slightly, with your hands placed on your thigh, and then move in the opposite direction.

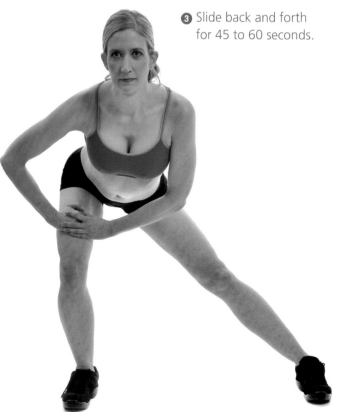

3 Slide back and forth for 45 to 60 seconds.

TARGETS
• Quadriceps
• Glutes
• Hamstrings

LEVEL
• Beginner

BENEFITS
• Strengthens and defines leg muscles

NOT ADVISABLE IF YOU HAVE . . .
• Hip issues
• Knee pain

DO IT RIGHT
• Push through the heel to drive the exercise.
• Move with control, keeping a steady, quick pace.

AVOID
• Hyperextending your knee past your toes.

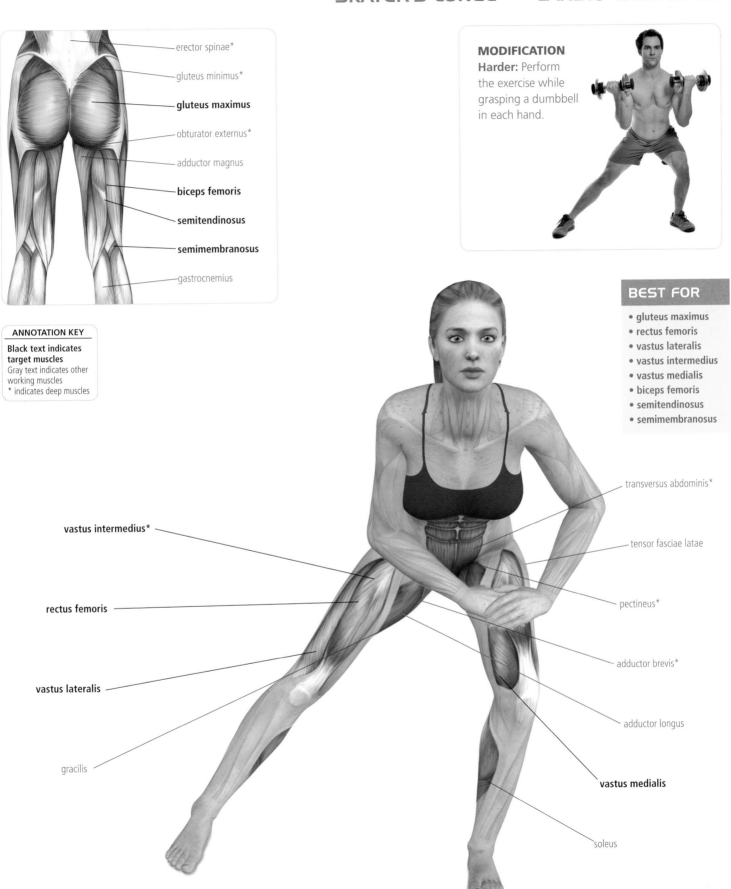

erector spinae*

gluteus minimus*

gluteus maximus

obturator externus*

adductor magnus

biceps femoris

semitendinosus

semimembranosus

gastrocnemius

ANNOTATION KEY

Black text indicates target muscles
Gray text indicates other working muscles
* indicates deep muscles

MODIFICATION
Harder: Perform the exercise while grasping a dumbbell in each hand.

BEST FOR

- **gluteus maximus**
- **rectus femoris**
- **vastus lateralis**
- **vastus intermedius**
- **vastus medialis**
- **biceps femoris**
- **semitendinosus**
- **semimembranosus**

vastus intermedius*

rectus femoris

vastus lateralis

gracilis

transversus abdominis*

tensor fasciae latae

pectineus*

adductor brevis*

adductor longus

vastus medialis

soleus

LATERAL STEPOVER

① Stand next to a flat bench.

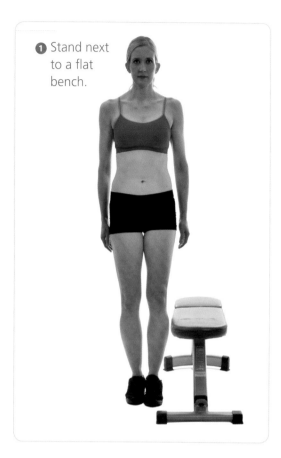

② Raise the knee of the leg closest to the bench, and then lower it down on the opposite side of the bench.

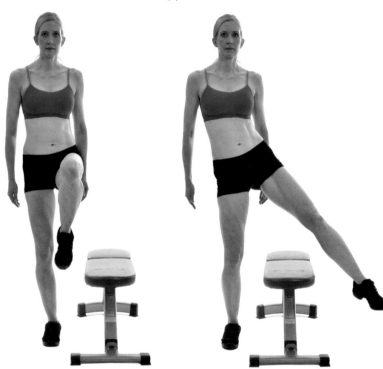

③ Lift the opposite leg to meet the other, bringing your feet together.

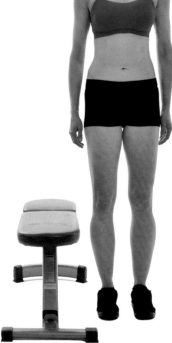

TARGETS
• Quadriceps
• Glutes
• Hamstrings

LEVEL
• Beginner

BENEFITS
• Strengthens leg muscles
• Builds endurance

NOT ADVISABLE IF YOU HAVE . . .
• Hip issues

BEST FOR

• gluteus maximus
• rectus femoris
• vastus lateralis
• vastus intermedius
• vastus medialis
• biceps femoris
• semitendinosus
• semimembranosus

AVOID
• Excessive speed.
• Sloppy form.
• Allowing your knees to hyperextend past your feet.

DO IT RIGHT
• Maintain a steady, even, but modest pace.
• Push through your heel to drive the movement.

4 Reverse the motion until you are standing with both feet together in the starting position. Continue for 15 to 20 complete repetitions.

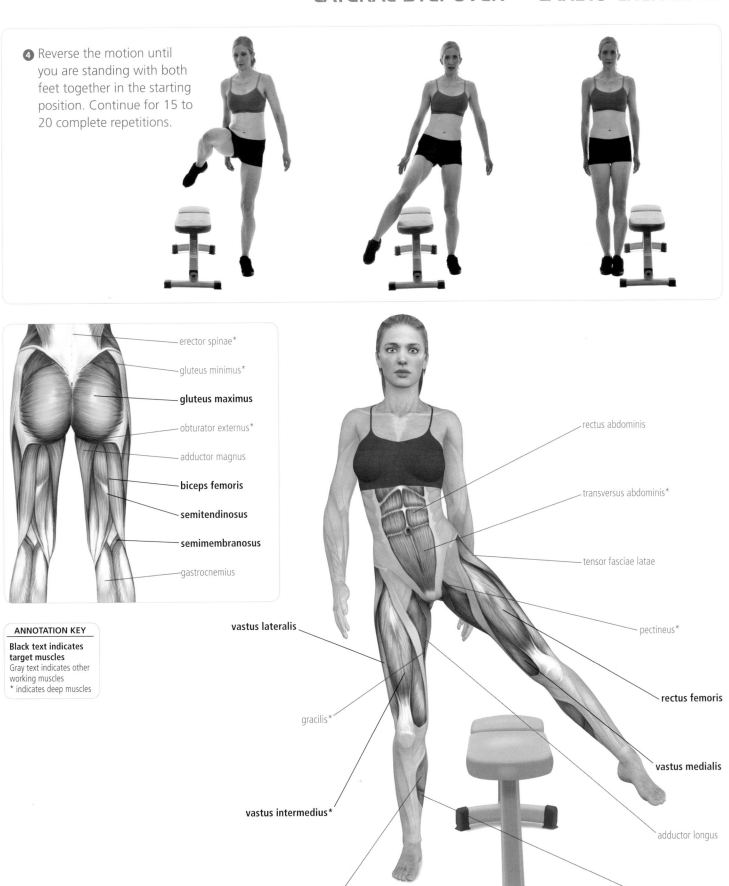

erector spinae*

gluteus minimus*

gluteus maximus

obturator externus*

adductor magnus

biceps femoris

semitendinosus

semimembranosus

gastrocnemius

ANNOTATION KEY

Black text indicates target muscles
Gray text indicates other working muscles
* indicates deep muscles

rectus abdominis

transversus abdominis*

tensor fasciae latae

pectineus*

rectus femoris

vastus medialis

adductor longus

soleus

vastus lateralis

gracilis*

vastus intermedius*

gastrocnemius

FLUTTER KICK

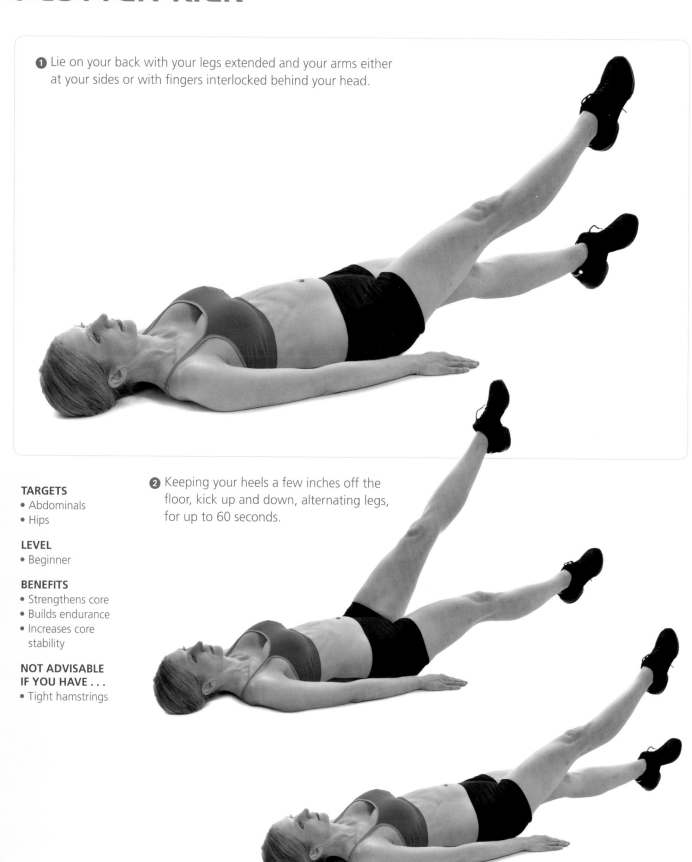

❶ Lie on your back with your legs extended and your arms either at your sides or with fingers interlocked behind your head.

TARGETS
• Abdominals
• Hips

LEVEL
• Beginner

BENEFITS
• Strengthens core
• Builds endurance
• Increases core stability

NOT ADVISABLE IF YOU HAVE . . .
• Tight hamstrings

❷ Keeping your heels a few inches off the floor, kick up and down, alternating legs, for up to 60 seconds.

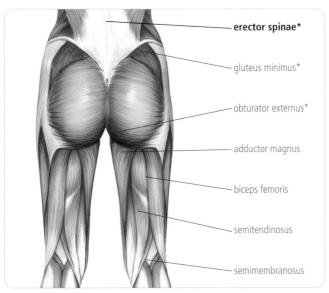

- erector spinae*
- gluteus minimus*
- obturator externus*
- adductor magnus
- biceps femoris
- semitendinosus
- semimembranosus

ANNOTATION KEY

Black text indicates target muscles
Gray text indicates other working muscles
* indicates deep muscles

AVOID
- Using momentum to drive the movement—keep a steady, moderate pace.
- Lifting your buttocks off the floor.

DO IT RIGHT
- Keep your legs as straight as possible.
- Draw your navel into your spine.

BEST FOR
- rectus abdominis
- obliquus externus
- obliquus internus
- erector spinae
- rectus femoris
- iliopsoas
- sartorius

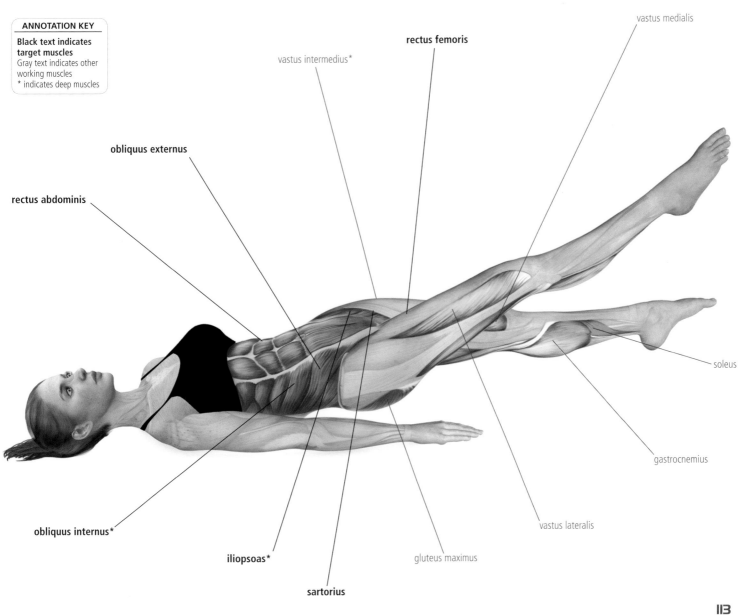

vastus medialis

rectus femoris

vastus intermedius*

obliquus externus

rectus abdominis

soleus

gastrocnemius

obliquus internus*

vastus lateralis

iliopsoas*

gluteus maximus

sartorius

POWER PUNCH

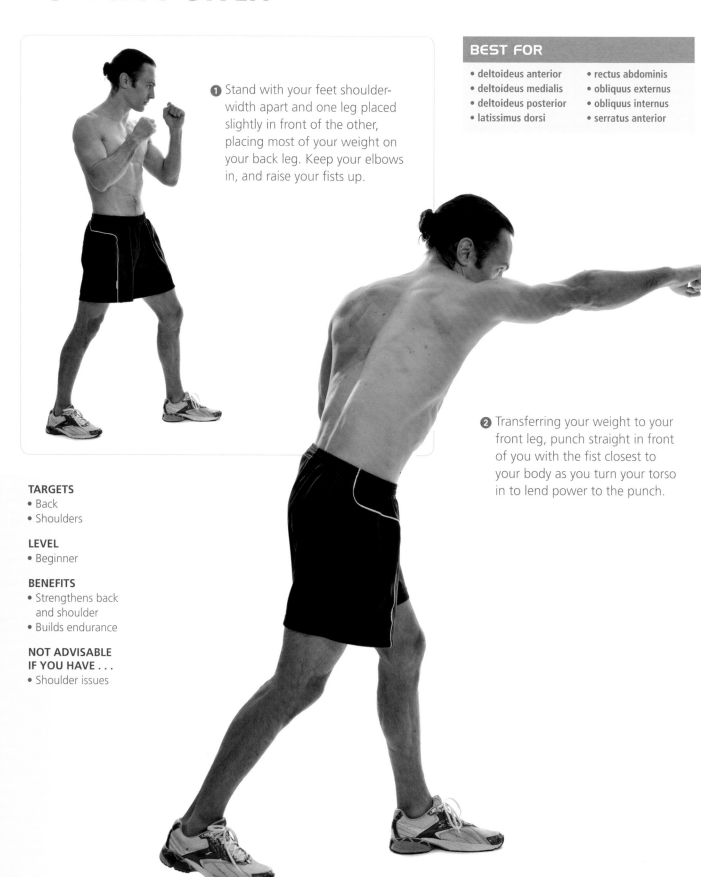

① Stand with your feet shoulder-width apart and one leg placed slightly in front of the other, placing most of your weight on your back leg. Keep your elbows in, and raise your fists up.

② Transferring your weight to your front leg, punch straight in front of you with the fist closest to your body as you turn your torso in to lend power to the punch.

TARGETS
- Back
- Shoulders

LEVEL
- Beginner

BENEFITS
- Strengthens back and shoulder
- Builds endurance

NOT ADVISABLE IF YOU HAVE . . .
- Shoulder issues

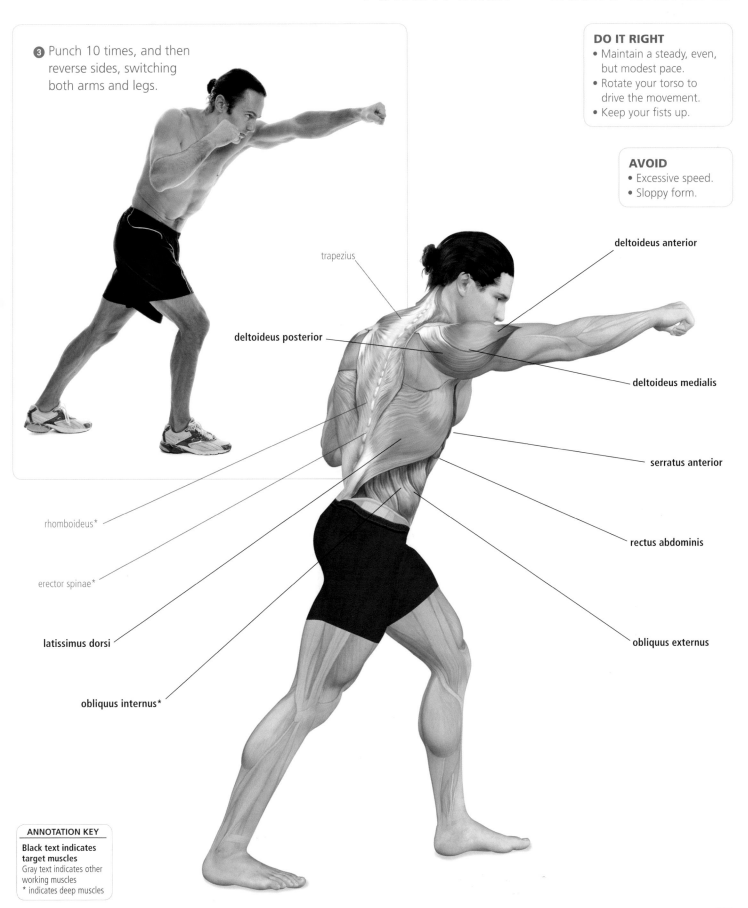

❸ Punch 10 times, and then reverse sides, switching both arms and legs.

DO IT RIGHT
- Maintain a steady, even, but modest pace.
- Rotate your torso to drive the movement.
- Keep your fists up.

AVOID
- Excessive speed.
- Sloppy form.

trapezius

deltoideus anterior

deltoideus posterior

deltoideus medialis

serratus anterior

rhomboideus*

rectus abdominis

erector spinae*

latissimus dorsi

obliquus externus

obliquus internus*

ANNOTATION KEY
Black text indicates target muscles
Gray text indicates other working muscles
* indicates deep muscles

UPPERCUT

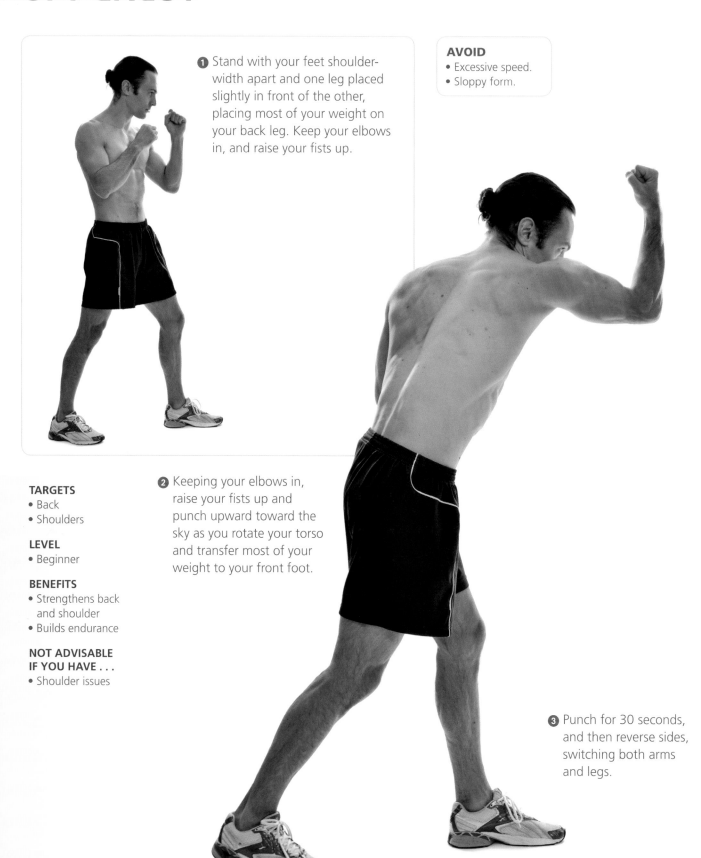

❶ Stand with your feet shoulder-width apart and one leg placed slightly in front of the other, placing most of your weight on your back leg. Keep your elbows in, and raise your fists up.

AVOID
• Excessive speed.
• Sloppy form.

TARGETS
• Back
• Shoulders

LEVEL
• Beginner

BENEFITS
• Strengthens back and shoulder
• Builds endurance

NOT ADVISABLE IF YOU HAVE . . .
• Shoulder issues

❷ Keeping your elbows in, raise your fists up and punch upward toward the sky as you rotate your torso and transfer most of your weight to your front foot.

❸ Punch for 30 seconds, and then reverse sides, switching both arms and legs.

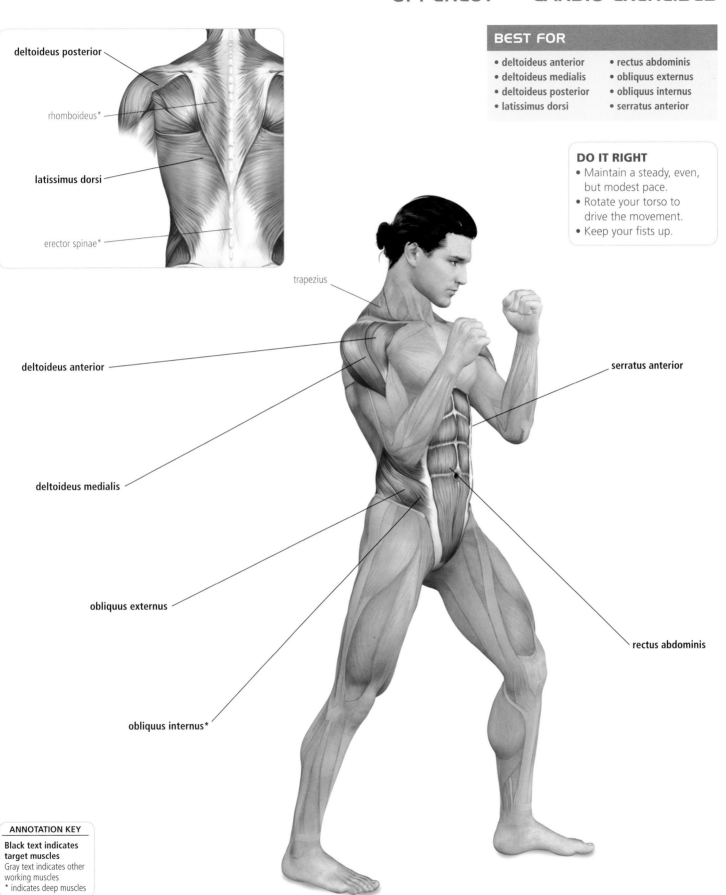

deltoideus posterior

rhomboideus*

latissimus dorsi

erector spinae*

trapezius

deltoideus anterior

deltoideus medialis

obliquus externus

obliquus internus*

serratus anterior

rectus abdominis

BEST FOR
- deltoideus anterior
- deltoideus medialis
- deltoideus posterior
- latissimus dorsi
- rectus abdominis
- obliquus externus
- obliquus internus
- serratus anterior

DO IT RIGHT
- Maintain a steady, even, but modest pace.
- Rotate your torso to drive the movement.
- Keep your fists up.

ANNOTATION KEY

Black text indicates target muscles
Gray text indicates other working muscles
* indicates deep muscles

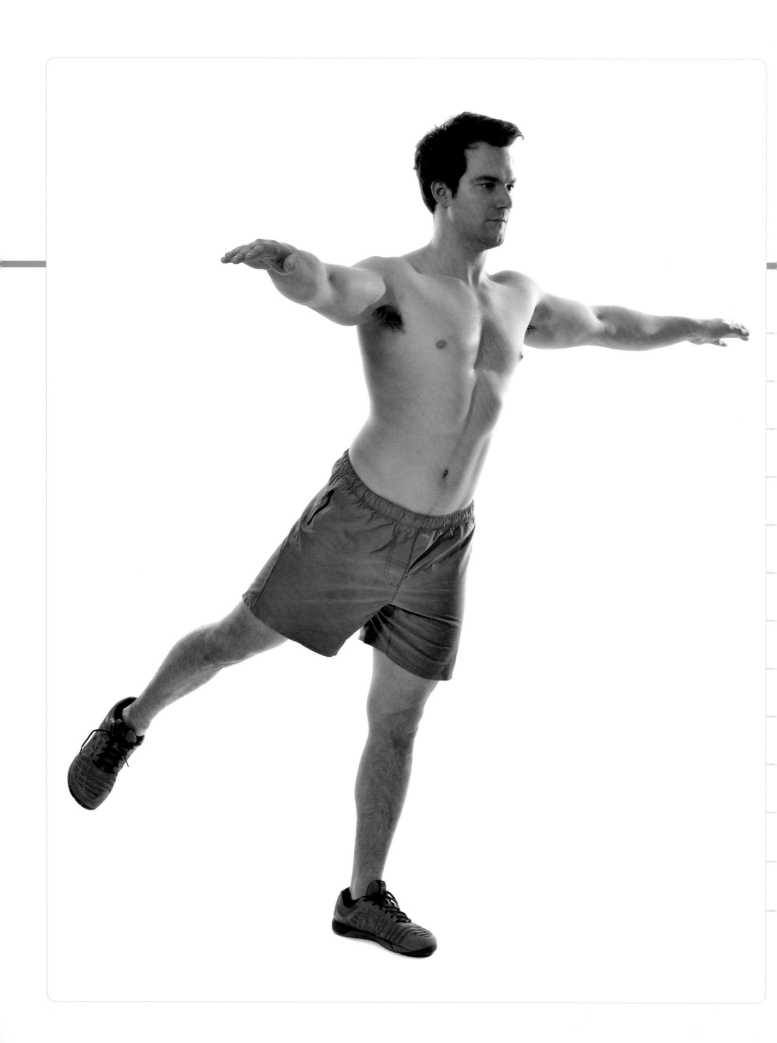

BALANCE EXERCISES

You can have ample strength, speed, stamina and even flexibility, but

without proper balance control, day-to-day movement will prove ineffective

and, perhaps, for some, nearly impossible. More than a third of us over the

age of 65 are likely to experience a fall at some point in our later years,

which can result in a serious hip injury or even worse. Performing regular

balance training, in addition to other modalities, will strengthen your

ability to maintain your body's natural position and help to prevent injuries,

whether you are in motion or even at rest.

STANDING ON ONE FOOT

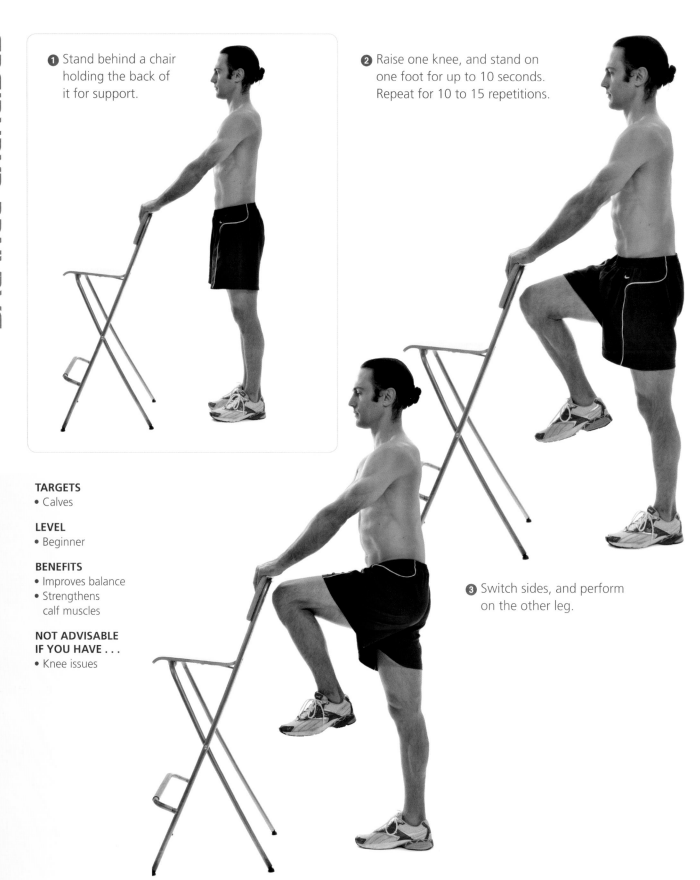

1 Stand behind a chair holding the back of it for support.

2 Raise one knee, and stand on one foot for up to 10 seconds. Repeat for 10 to 15 repetitions.

3 Switch sides, and perform on the other leg.

TARGETS
• Calves

LEVEL
• Beginner

BENEFITS
• Improves balance
• Strengthens calf muscles

NOT ADVISABLE IF YOU HAVE . . .
• Knee issues

MODIFICATION

Harder: Raise your arms to the sides, parallel to your shoulders.

DO IT RIGHT
- Keep your spine long.
- Maintain good posture throughout the exercise.

AVOID
- Slouching or rounding your back.
- Pushing through your toe instead of your heel.

erector spinae*

BEST FOR
- soleus
- gastrocnemius
- tibialis anterior

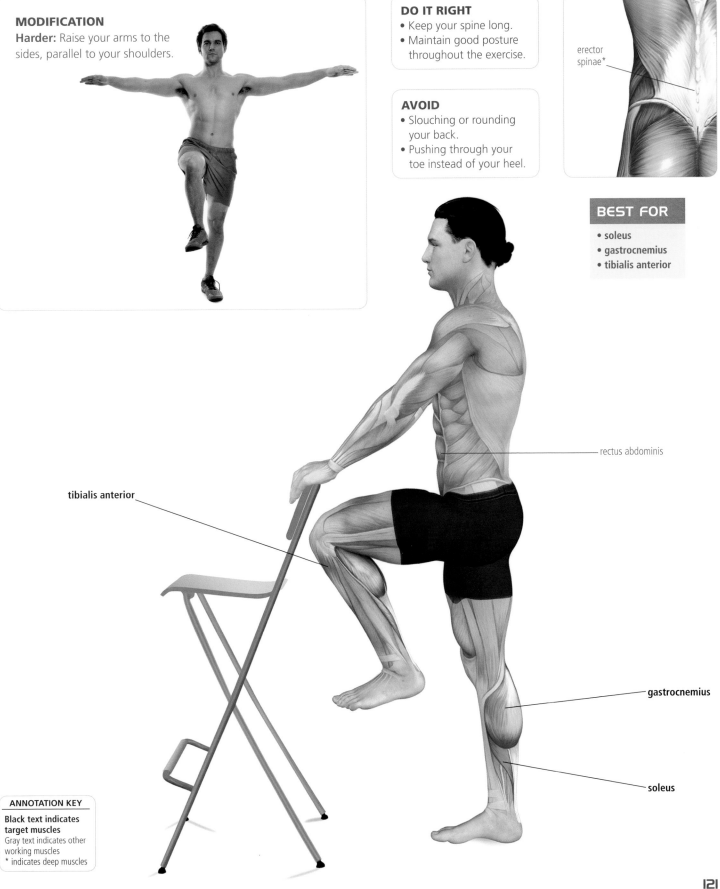

rectus abdominis

tibialis anterior

gastrocnemius

soleus

ANNOTATION KEY
Black text indicates target muscles
Gray text indicates other working muscles
* indicates deep muscles

WALKING HEEL-TO-TOE

① Begin standing while positioning the heel of one foot just past the toes of the other, while the two are just barely touching.

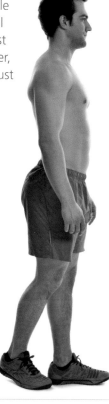

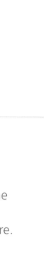

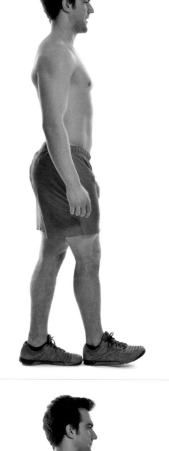

TARGETS
• Calves

LEVEL
• Beginner

BENEFITS
• Improves balance

NOT ADVISABLE IF YOU HAVE . . .
• Safe for most

② Choose a target that lies straight ahead, and place one foot repeatedly ahead of the other while walking a straight line to get there.

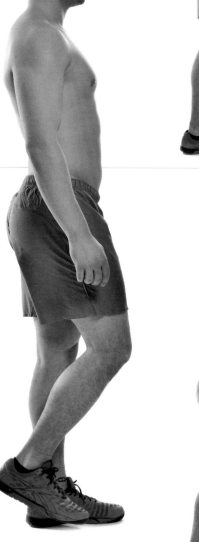

3 Continue walking heel-to-toe for a total of 20 steps.

DO IT RIGHT
- Keep your spine long.
- Maintain good posture throughout the exercise.

AVOID
- Slouching or rounding your back.
- Pushing through your toe instead of your heel.

erector spinae*

BEST FOR
- soleus
- gastrocnemius
- tibialis anterior

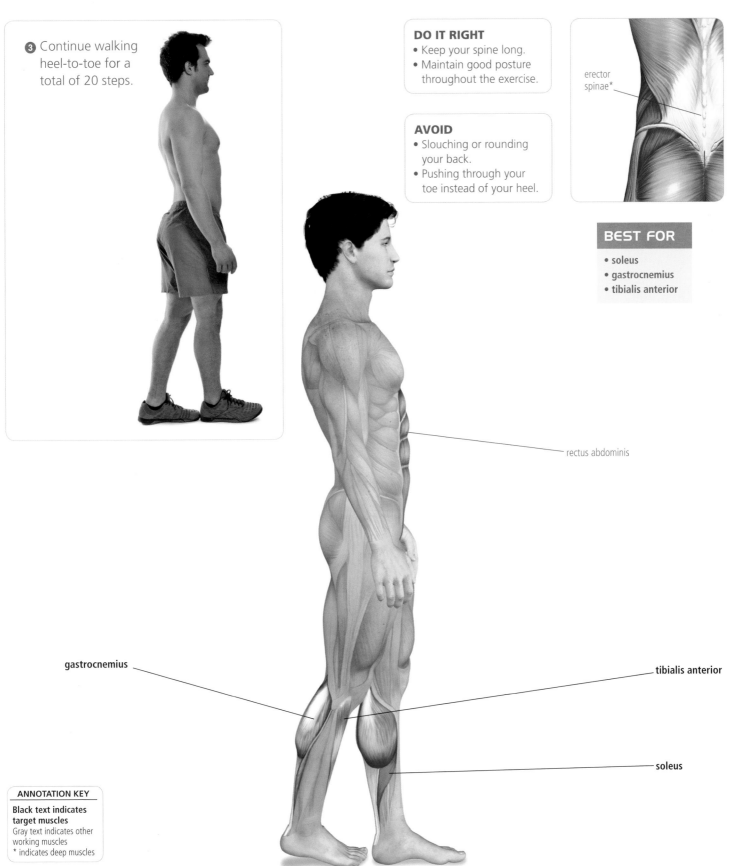

rectus abdominis

gastrocnemius

tibialis anterior

soleus

ANNOTATION KEY

Black text indicates target muscles
Gray text indicates other working muscles
* indicates deep muscles

BALANCE WALK

❶ Begin by raising your arms out to your sides at shoulder height.

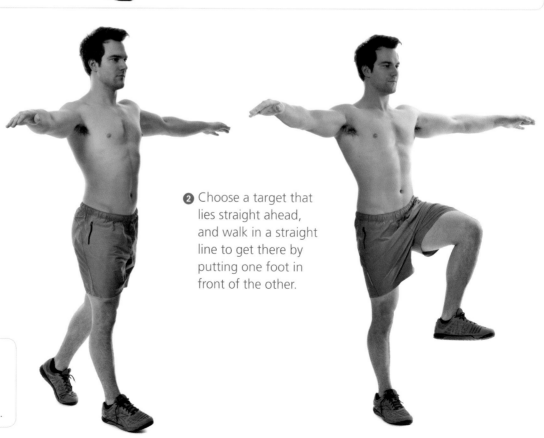

TARGETS
• Calves
• Shoulders

LEVEL
• Beginner

BENEFITS
• Improves balance

NOT ADVISABLE IF YOU HAVE . . .
• Inner-ear issues

❷ Choose a target that lies straight ahead, and walk in a straight line to get there by putting one foot in front of the other.

AVOID
• Slouching or rounding your back.
• Pushing through your toe instead of your heel.

3 Lift your back leg as you walk, and then pause for 1 second before continuing for 20 steps per leg.

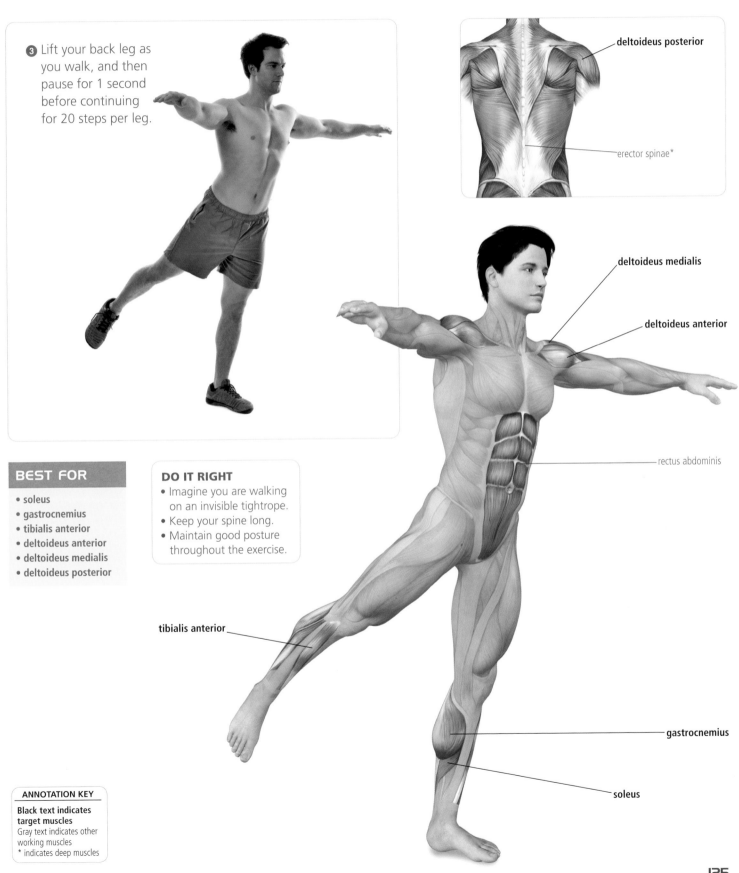

deltoideus posterior

erector spinae*

deltoideus medialis

deltoideus anterior

rectus abdominis

tibialis anterior

gastrocnemius

soleus

BEST FOR

- soleus
- gastrocnemius
- tibialis anterior
- deltoideus anterior
- deltoideus medialis
- deltoideus posterior

DO IT RIGHT

- Imagine you are walking on an invisible tightrope.
- Keep your spine long.
- Maintain good posture throughout the exercise.

ANNOTATION KEY

Black text indicates target muscles
Gray text indicates other working muscles
* indicates deep muscles

SWISS BALL ONE-ARM ROW

❶ Begin by standing in front of a Swiss ball with your right knee placed on the ball and your left foot on the floor. Place your right palm on the ball, while grasping a dumbbell in your left hand with your arm extended downward.

BEST FOR

• latissimus dorsi

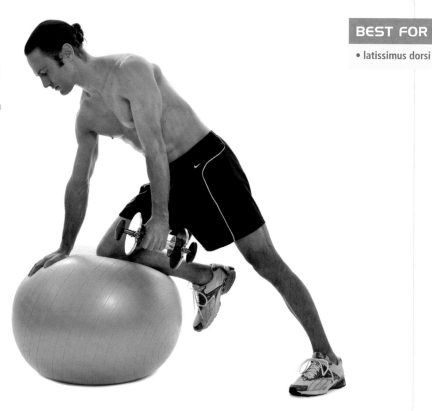

TARGETS
• Outer back

LEVEL
• Beginner

BENEFITS
• Strengthens the outer back
• Stabilizes core

NOT ADVISABLE IF YOU HAVE . . .
• Shoulder issues
• Lower-back pain

❷ Maintain a flat back as you pull the dumbbell up next to your chest, strongly contracting the latissimus dorsi muscle in your back.

AVOID
• Excessive speed or momentum.
• Rounding your back.

DO IT RIGHT
• Maintain a flat back throughout the movement.
• Pull toward your chest.

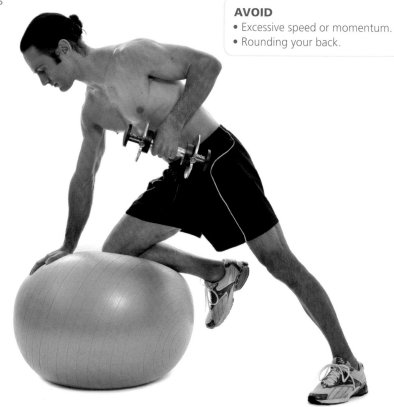

3 Lower the dumbbell back down to full extension, and then repeat the exercise for 12 to 15 repetitions. Switch sides, and repeat with your right arm.

brachioradialis

extensor carpi radialis longus

extensor carpi ulnaris

extensor digitorum

extensor carpi radialis brevis

extensor digiti minimi

flexor carpi ulnaris

abductor pollicis longus

extensor pollicis brevis

rhomboideus*

erector spinae*

deltoideus posterior

biceps brachii

latissimus dorsi

rectus abdominis

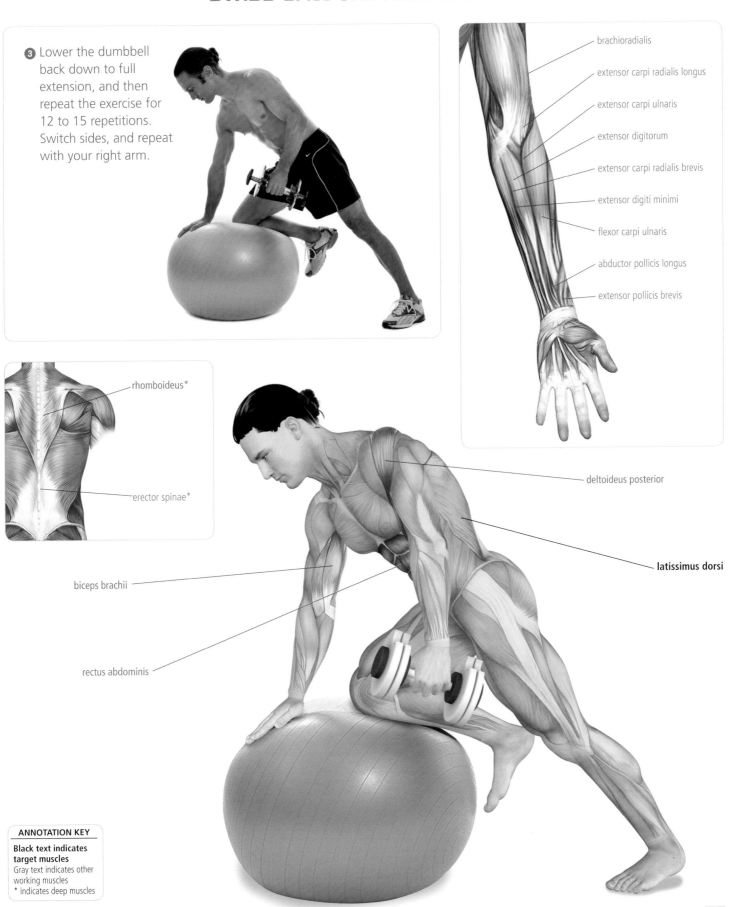

ANNOTATION KEY

Black text indicates target muscles
Gray text indicates other working muscles
* indicates deep muscles

SINGLE-LEG DEADLIFT

1 Begin in a standing position holding a pair of dumbbells and maintaining a soft knee while keeping the opposite leg slightly bent and elevated above the floor.

BEST FOR

- biceps femoris
- semitendinosus
- semimembranosus
- gluteus maximus
- adductor magnus

AVOID

- Lowering the weights beyond a mild stretch through the hamstrings.
- Rounding your back.
- Excessive speed or momentum.

DO IT RIGHT

- Maintain a full range of motion.
- Keep your knees soft throughout the movement.

TARGETS
- Glutes
- Hamstrings

LEVEL
- Beginner/ Intermediate

BENEFITS
- Strengthens glutes and hamstrings

NOT ADVISABLE IF YOU HAVE . . .
- Hamstring injury
- Shoulder issues
- Wrist issues

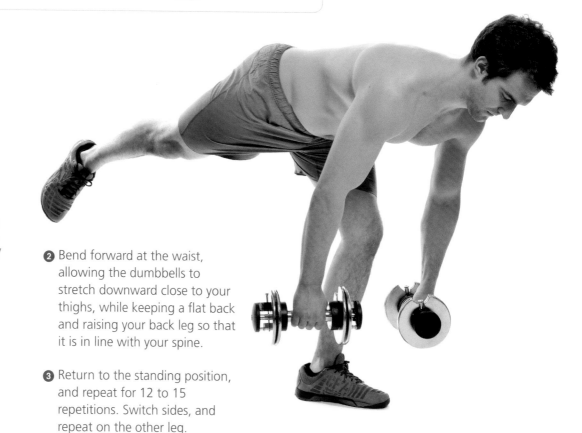

2 Bend forward at the waist, allowing the dumbbells to stretch downward close to your thighs, while keeping a flat back and raising your back leg so that it is in line with your spine.

3 Return to the standing position, and repeat for 12 to 15 repetitions. Switch sides, and repeat on the other leg.

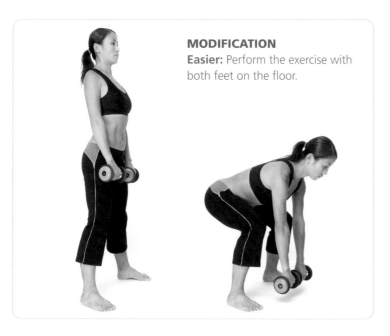

MODIFICATION

Easier: Perform the exercise with both feet on the floor.

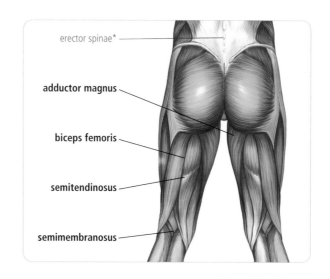

erector spinae*

adductor magnus

biceps femoris

semitendinosus

semimembranosus

ANNOTATION KEY

Black text indicates target muscles
Gray text indicates other working muscles
* indicates deep muscles

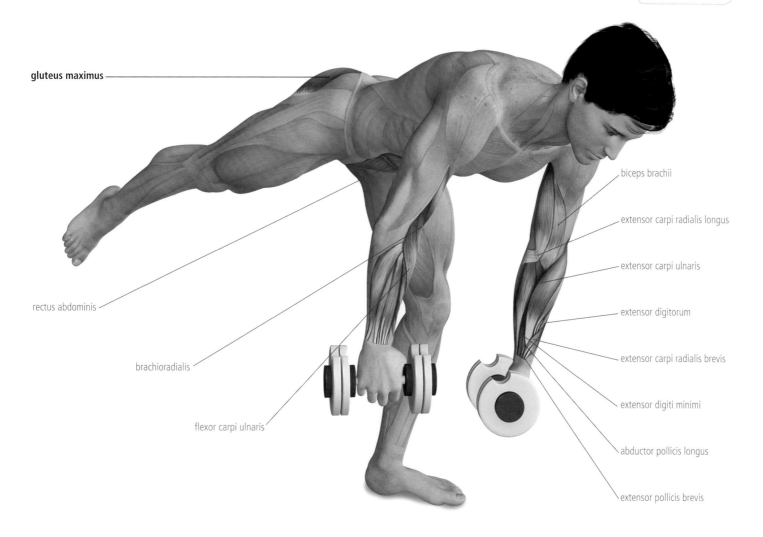

gluteus maximus

biceps brachii

extensor carpi radialis longus

extensor carpi ulnaris

extensor digitorum

extensor carpi radialis brevis

rectus abdominis

extensor digiti minimi

brachioradialis

abductor pollicis longus

flexor carpi ulnaris

extensor pollicis brevis

SWISS BALL HAMSTRING FLEXIBILITY

1. Begin standing on one foot with the other leg outstretched and placed on a Swiss-Ball to your side.

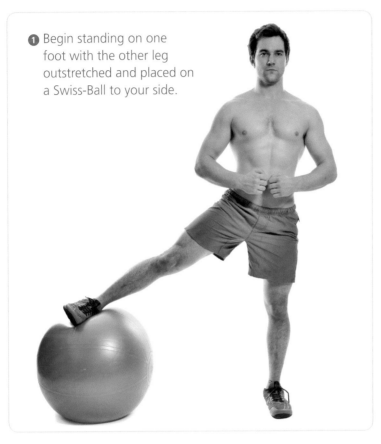

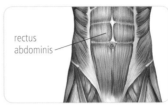

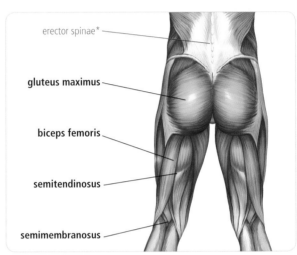

rectus abdominis

erector spinae*

gluteus maximus

biceps femoris

semitendinosus

semimembranosus

BEST FOR

- **gluteus maximus**
- **biceps femoris**
- **semitendinosus**
- **semimembranosus**

DO IT RIGHT
- Keep your abdominals braced.
- Maintain soft knees.

ANNOTATION KEY
Black text indicates target muscles
Gray text indicates other working muscles
* indicates deep muscles

TARGETS
- Hamstrings
- Glutes

LEVEL
- Beginner

BENEFITS
- Stretches hamstrings and gluteals
- Promotes better balance

NOT ADVISABLE IF YOU HAVE . . .
- Hamstring injury

2. While keeping the supported knee soft and your abdominals braced, bend toward your knee and hold for 20 to 30 seconds. Switch sides, and repeat.

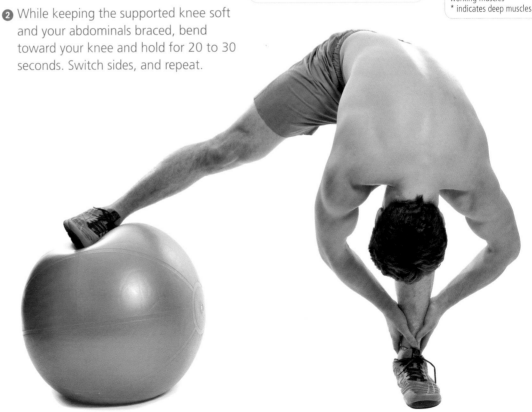

AVOID
- Excessive speed.
- Bouncy repetitions.

SITTING BALANCE

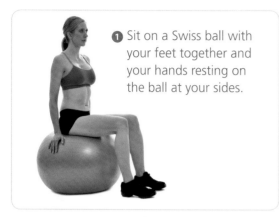

❶ Sit on a Swiss ball with your feet together and your hands resting on the ball at your sides.

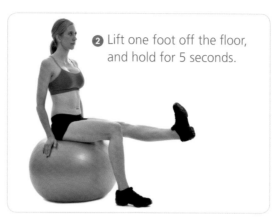

❷ Lift one foot off the floor, and hold for 5 seconds.

BEST FOR

- rectus abdominis
- rectus femoris
- vastus lateralis
- vastus intermedius
- vastus medialis

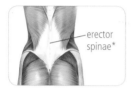

iliopsoas*

pectineus*

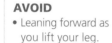

erector spinae*

ANNOTATION KEY

Black text indicates target muscles
Gray text indicates other working muscles
* indicates deep muscles

AVOID

- Leaning forward as you lift your leg.

❸ Put your foot down, and then lift your other foot. Repeat five times on each leg.

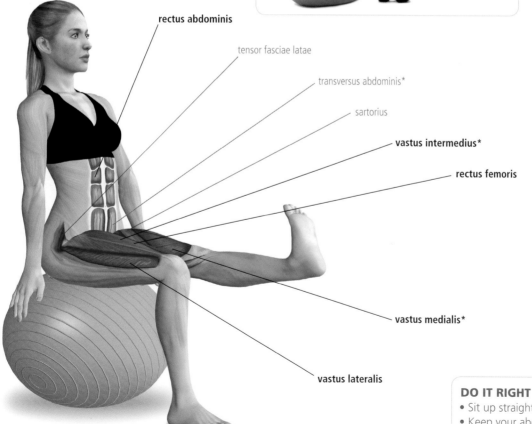

rectus abdominis

tensor fasciae latae

transversus abdominis*

sartorius

vastus intermedius*

rectus femoris

vastus medialis*

vastus lateralis

TARGETS

- Abdominals
- Quadriceps

LEVEL

- Beginner

BENEFITS

- Stabilizes core
- Strengthens abdominals

NOT ADVISABLE IF YOU HAVE . . .

- Neck issues
- Lower-back pain

DO IT RIGHT

- Sit up straight.
- Keep your abdominals activated.

SWISS BALL PLANK WITH LEG RAISE

① Begin in a prone position balanced on your toes with your forearms planted on a Swiss ball.

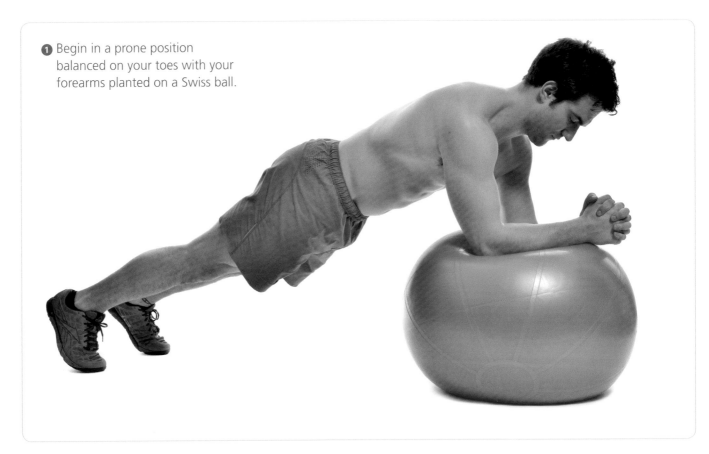

TARGETS
• Core

LEVEL
• Intermediate

BENEFITS
• Strengthens core

NOT ADVISABLE IF YOU HAVE . . .
• Shoulder instability
• Lower-back pain

② Slowly raise one leg from the floor while keeping your spine in one straight line.

③ Hold for 10 to 30 seconds, and then repeat with the other leg.

MODIFICATION

Easier: Maintain the prone position balanced on your toes with your forearms planted on the Swiss ball for 30 seconds.

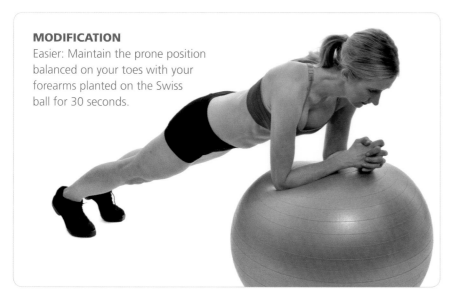

DO IT RIGHT
• Maintain a neutral spine alignment.

AVOID
• Allowing your spine to arch or sag.

BEST FOR
• erector spinae
• rectus abdominis

ANNOTATION KEY

Black text indicates target muscles
Gray text indicates other working muscles
* indicates deep muscles

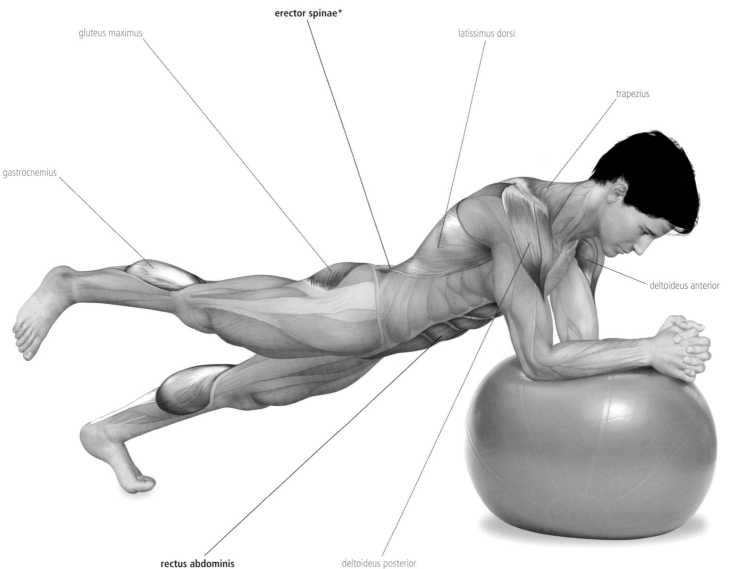

gluteus maximus

erector spinae*

latissimus dorsi

trapezius

gastrocnemius

deltoideus anterior

rectus abdominis

deltoideus posterior

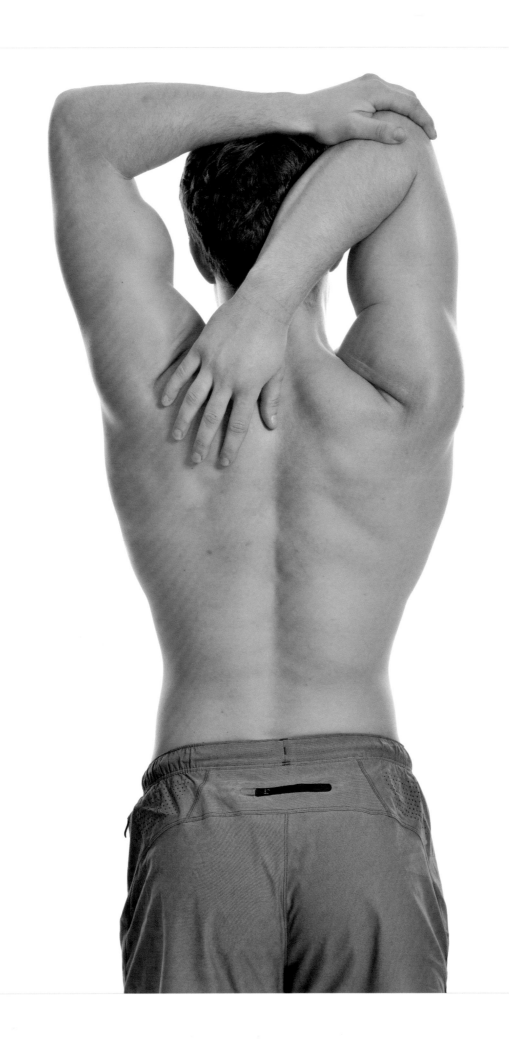

FLEXIBILITY STRETCHES

Stretching serves as an effective intra-workout modality, and it also burns calories, as well as helps to elevate the metabolism. This kind of exercise further allows a joint and muscle to work through a full range of motion. Stretching and flexibility can also lead to a decrease in injuries by allowing improved blood flow and muscle relaxation. Controlled elongation through a muscle can mean less pain and an increase in your overall health, vitality and even promote tranquility. For a form of exercise that takes mere minutes a day to complete, the benefits are just too great to neglect, so make flexibility stretches a permanent part of your longevity regimen.

SEATED LEG CRADLE

1 Sit on the floor with your legs extended in front of you.

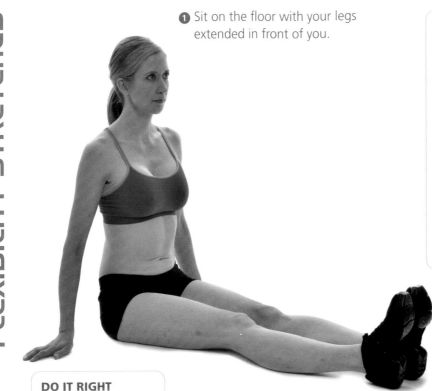

gluteus medius*

gluteus minimus*

gluteus maximus

piriformis*

biceps femoris

semitendinosus

semimembranosus

ANNOTATION KEY

Black text indicates target muscles
Gray text indicates other working muscles
* indicates deep muscles

BEST FOR

• biceps femoris
• semitendinosus
• semimembranosus
• gluteus maximus

DO IT RIGHT
• Fully contract your gluteal muscles.

TARGETS
• Glutes
• Hamstrings

LEVEL
• Beginner

BENEFITS
• Stretches glutes and hamstrings

NOT ADVISABLE IF YOU HAVE . . .
• Hip issues
• Knee pain

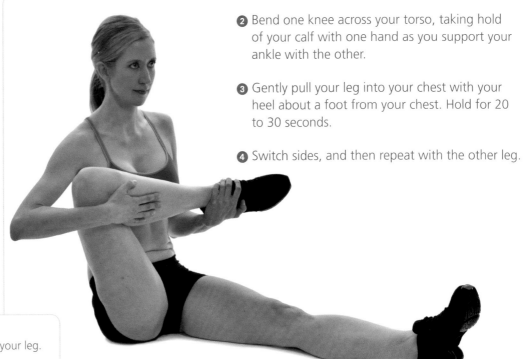

2 Bend one knee across your torso, taking hold of your calf with one hand as you support your ankle with the other.

3 Gently pull your leg into your chest with your heel about a foot from your chest. Hold for 20 to 30 seconds.

4 Switch sides, and then repeat with the other leg.

AVOID
• Aggressively pulling on your leg.
• Holding your breath.

BUTTERFLY STRETCH

1. Sit up tall on the floor or a mat, with the soles of your feet pressed together.

2. Place your forearms or elbows on your inner thighs, and grab your feet and toes with your hands.

3. Draw your heels in toward your core.

4. Hold for 15 to 30 seconds.

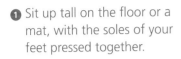

BEST FOR

- adductor longus
- adductor magnus
- adductor brevis

pectineus*

adductor longus

adductor brevis*

gracilis

ANNOTATION KEY

Black text indicates target muscles
Gray text indicates other working muscles
* indicates deep muscles

TARGETS
- Adductors
- Lower back

LEVEL
- Beginner

BENEFITS
- Stretches inner thighs and lower back

NOT ADVISABLE IF YOU HAVE . . .
- Hip issues
- Knee pain

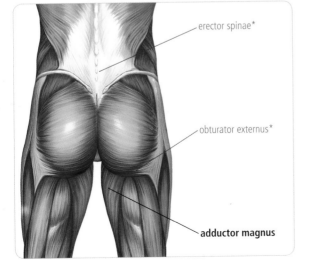

erector spinae*

obturator externus*

adductor magnus

DO IT RIGHT
- Do not compromise the position of your upper body: sit nice and tall, and try to feel your hip bones on the floor.

AVOID
- Holding your breath.
- Rocking backward, off your hip bones; instead, feel them anchored on the floor.

HIP AND LOWER-BACK STRETCH

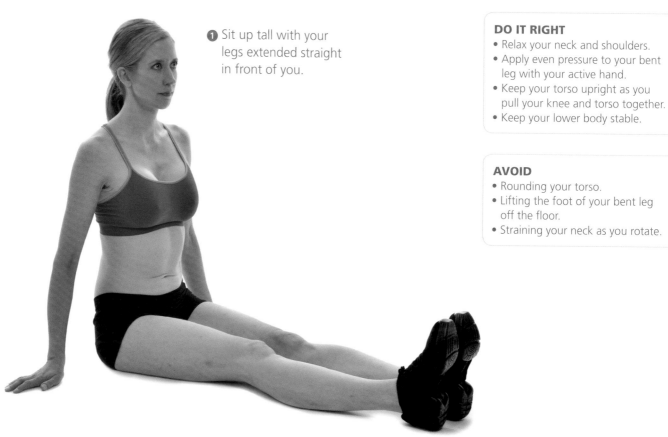

① Sit up tall with your legs extended straight in front of you.

DO IT RIGHT
- Relax your neck and shoulders.
- Apply even pressure to your bent leg with your active hand.
- Keep your torso upright as you pull your knee and torso together.
- Keep your lower body stable.

AVOID
- Rounding your torso.
- Lifting the foot of your bent leg off the floor.
- Straining your neck as you rotate.

TARGETS
- Hips
- Gluteal muscles
- Spine
- Obliques

LEVEL
- Intermediate

BENEFITS
- Stretches hip extensors and flexors
- Stretches obliques and latissimus dorsi

NOT ADVISABLE IF YOU HAVE . . .
- Hip dysfunction
- Severe lower-back pain

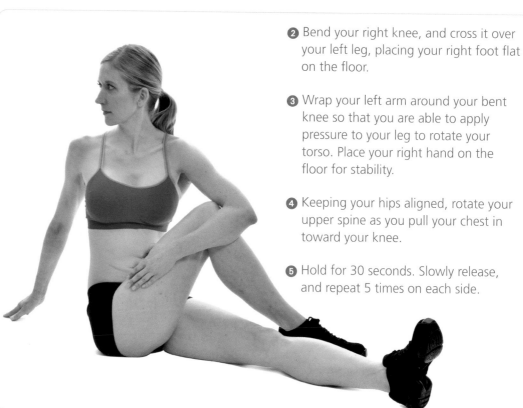

② Bend your right knee, and cross it over your left leg, placing your right foot flat on the floor.

③ Wrap your left arm around your bent knee so that you are able to apply pressure to your leg to rotate your torso. Place your right hand on the floor for stability.

④ Keeping your hips aligned, rotate your upper spine as you pull your chest in toward your knee.

⑤ Hold for 30 seconds. Slowly release, and repeat 5 times on each side.

BEST FOR

- adductor longus
- iliopsoas
- rhomboideus
- sternocleidomastoideus
- obliquus externus
- obliquus internus
- latissimus dorsi
- multifidus spinae
- erector spinae
- tractus iliotibialis
- gluteus maximus
- gluteus medius
- piriformis

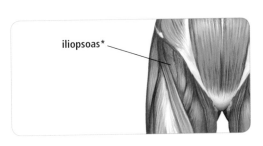

iliopsoas*

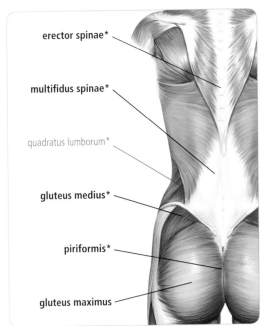

erector spinae*

multifidus spinae*

quadratus lumborum*

gluteus medius*

piriformis*

gluteus maximus

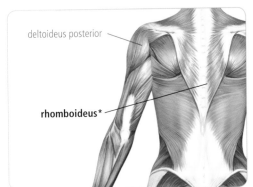

deltoideus posterior

rhomboideus*

ANNOTATION KEY

Black text indicates target muscles
Gray text indicates other working muscles
* indicates deep muscles

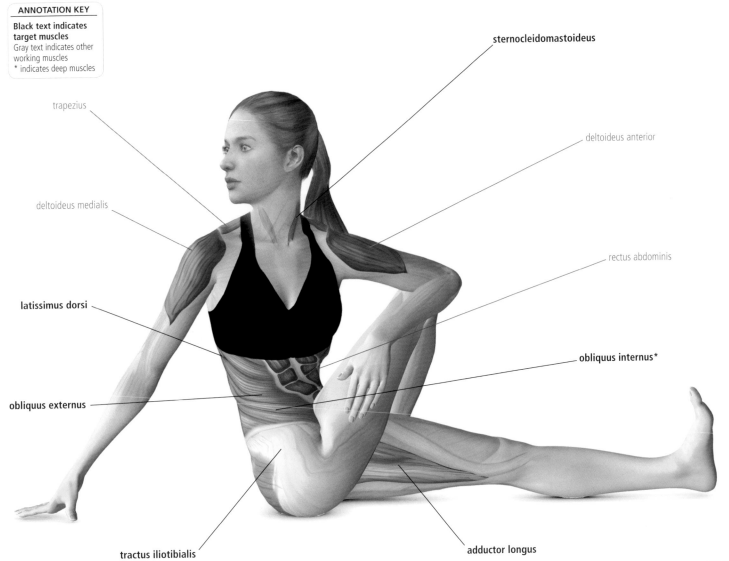

trapezius

deltoideus medialis

latissimus dorsi

obliquus externus

tractus iliotibialis

sternocleidomastoideus

deltoideus anterior

rectus abdominis

obliquus internus*

adductor longus

SIDE-LYING KNEE BEND

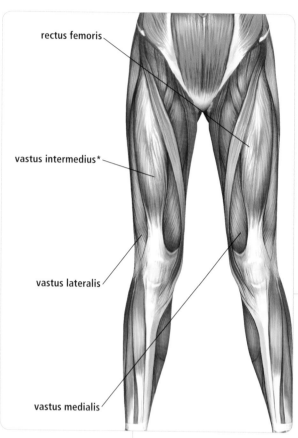

rectus femoris

vastus intermedius*

vastus lateralis

vastus medialis

BEST FOR

- rectus femoris
- vastus lateralis
- vastus intermedius
- vastus medialis

ANNOTATION KEY

Black text indicates target muscles
Gray text indicates other working muscles
* indicates deep muscles

DO IT RIGHT

- Keep your knees together, one on top of the other.
- Tuck your pelvis slightly forward, and lift your chest to fully engage and stretch your core.
- Keep your bottom foot pointed and parallel with your leg.

AVOID

- Leaning back onto your gluteal muscles.

❶ Lie on your left side, with your legs extended together in line with your body. Extend your left arm, and rest your head on your upper arm.

TARGETS
- Quadriceps

LEVEL
- Beginner

BENEFITS
- Stretches thigh muscles

NOT ADVISABLE IF YOU HAVE . . .
- Knee issues

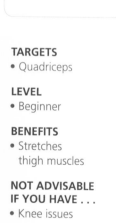

❷ Bend your right knee and grasp the ankle with your right hand.

❸ Pull your ankle in toward your buttocks as you stretch. Hold for 10 to 30 seconds.

❹ Return to the starting position, and repeat on the other side.

KNEELING LAT STRETCH

1 Begin kneeling with your thighs resting on your ankles, your torso elongated forward and your arms extended in front of you with your forehead resting on the floor and your palms facing downward.

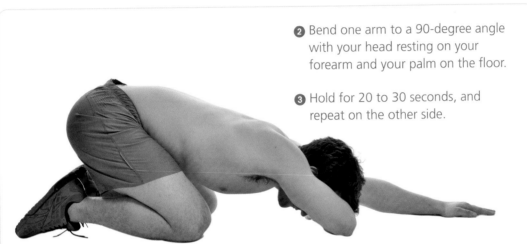

BEST FOR

- **latissimus dorsi**
- **rectus femoris**
- **vastus lateralis**
- **vastus intermedius**
- **vastus medialis**

DO IT RIGHT
- Fully elongate your back, feeling a complete stretch.

AVOID
- Hyperextending your back.

2 Bend one arm to a 90-degree angle with your head resting on your forearm and your palm on the floor.

3 Hold for 20 to 30 seconds, and repeat on the other side.

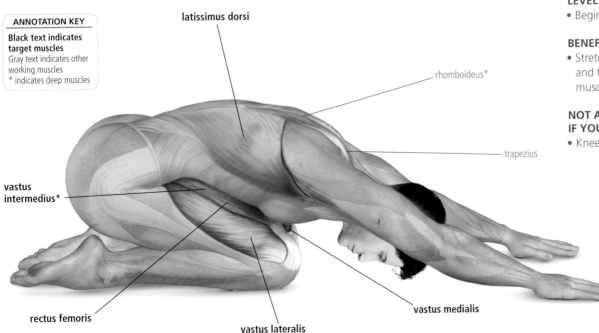

TARGETS
- Back
- Quadriceps

LEVEL
- Beginner

BENEFITS
- Stretches back and thigh muscles

NOT ADVISABLE IF YOU HAVE . . .
- Knee issues

ANNOTATION KEY

Black text indicates target muscles
Gray text indicates other working muscles
* indicates deep muscles

latissimus dorsi

rhomboideus*

trapezius

vastus intermedius*

rectus femoris

vastus lateralis

vastus medialis

TRICEPS STRETCH

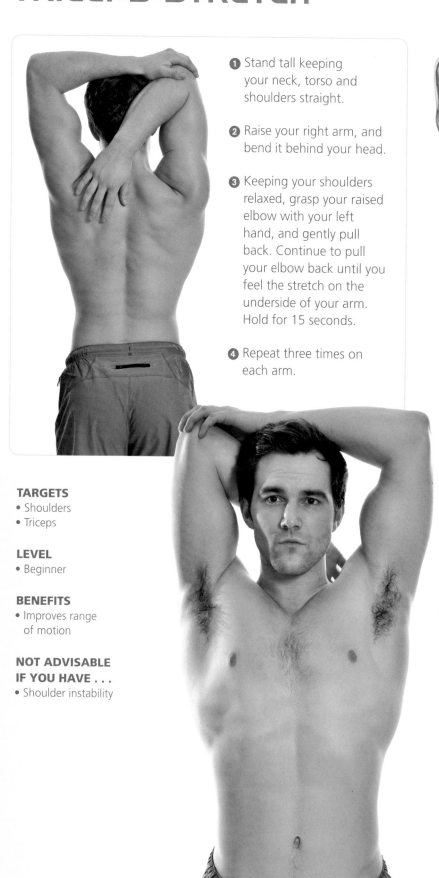

1. Stand tall keeping your neck, torso and shoulders straight.

2. Raise your right arm, and bend it behind your head.

3. Keeping your shoulders relaxed, grasp your raised elbow with your left hand, and gently pull back. Continue to pull your elbow back until you feel the stretch on the underside of your arm. Hold for 15 seconds.

4. Repeat three times on each arm.

triceps brachii

deltoideus posterior

ANNOTATION KEY

Black text indicates target muscles
Gray text indicates other working muscles
* indicates deep muscles

TARGETS
• Shoulders
• Triceps

LEVEL
• Beginner

BENEFITS
• Improves range of motion

NOT ADVISABLE IF YOU HAVE . . .
• Shoulder instability

BEST FOR

• triceps brachii
• deltoideus posterior

AVOID
• Leaning backward.

DO IT RIGHT
• Keep your dropped elbow close to the side of your head.

BICEPS STRETCH

① Begin in a standing position with your feet shoulder-width apart and your knees kept soft.

② Clasp your hands together behind your back as you straighten your arms downward, while simultaneously twisting your palms inward to feel the stretch. Hold for 20 to 30 seconds.

DO IT RIGHT
• Keep your shoulders pressed downward and back.

BEST FOR
• pectoralis major
• pectoralis minor
• biceps brachii

ANNOTATION KEY

Black text indicates target muscles
Gray text indicates other working muscles
* indicates deep muscles

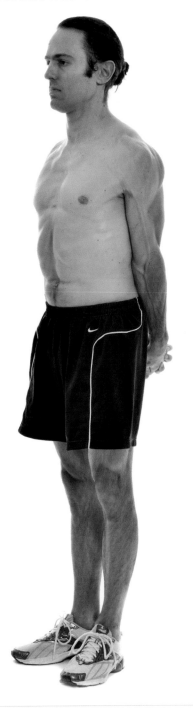

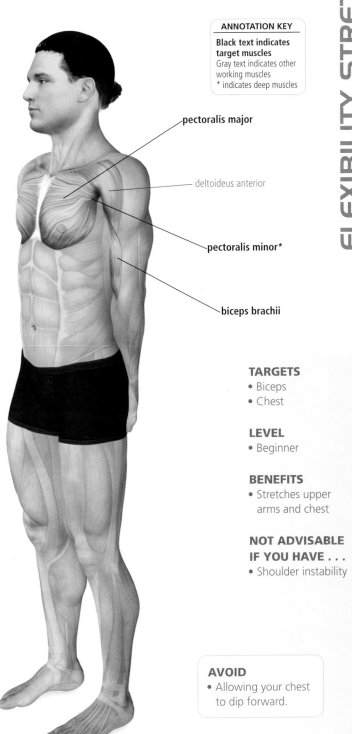

pectoralis major

deltoideus anterior

pectoralis minor*

biceps brachii

TARGETS
• Biceps
• Chest

LEVEL
• Beginner

BENEFITS
• Stretches upper arms and chest

NOT ADVISABLE IF YOU HAVE . . .
• Shoulder instability

AVOID
• Allowing your chest to dip forward.

WALL-ASSISTED CHEST STRETCH

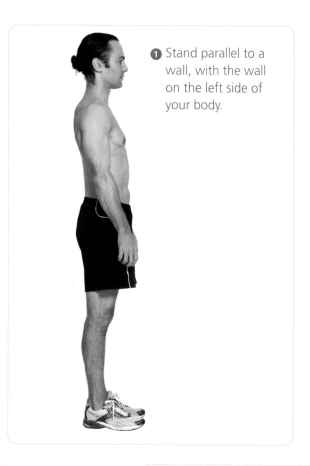

❶ Stand parallel to a wall, with the wall on the left side of your body.

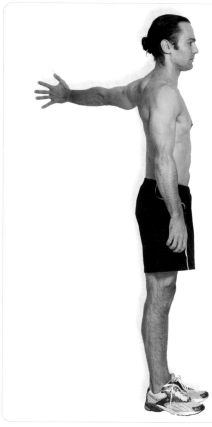

❷ Extend your left arm back against the wall, so that your palm is flat against it.

TARGETS
• Chest

LEVEL
• Beginner

BENEFITS
• Stretches the pectoral muscles

NOT ADVISABLE IF YOU HAVE . . .
• Shoulder issues

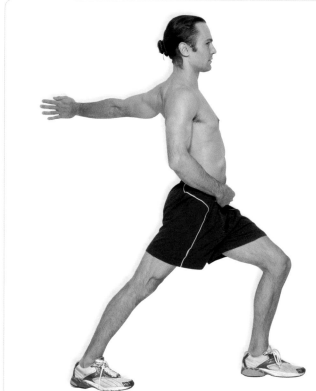

❸ Lunge forward with your left foot.

❹ Remain facing forward as you stretch. To stay aware of any torso twisting, place your right hand just below your left pectoral muscle, fingers on your rib cage.

❺ Hold for 20 to 30 seconds, and then return to the starting position, turn so that the wall is on your right, and repeat.

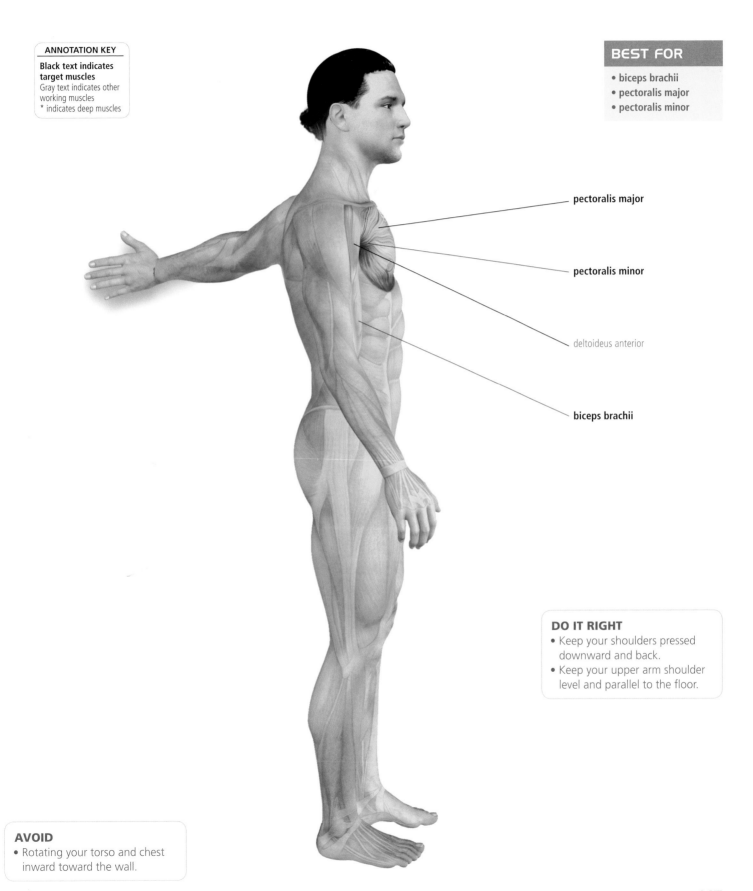

ANNOTATION KEY

Black text indicates target muscles
Gray text indicates other working muscles
* indicates deep muscles

BEST FOR

- biceps brachii
- pectoralis major
- pectoralis minor

pectoralis major

pectoralis minor

deltoideus anterior

biceps brachii

DO IT RIGHT
- Keep your shoulders pressed downward and back.
- Keep your upper arm shoulder level and parallel to the floor.

AVOID
- Rotating your torso and chest inward toward the wall.

SHOULDER STRETCH

BEST FOR

- deltoideus anterior
- pectoralis major
- pectoralis minor

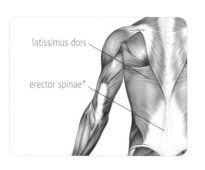

latissimus dors

erector spinae*

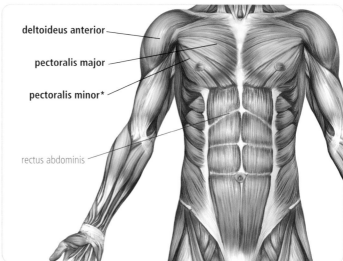

deltoideus anterior

pectoralis major

pectoralis minor*

rectus abdominis

ANNOTATION KEY

Black text indicates target muscles
Gray text indicates other working muscles
* indicates deep muscles

AVOID
- Shrugging your stretched shoulder upward—keep it roughly in line with your opposite arm's wrist.

DO IT RIGHT
- Keep your spine vertical and your lengthened arm firmly across your torso.

TARGETS
- Shoulders

LEVEL
- Beginner

BENEFITS
- Increases shoulder mobility

NOT ADVISABLE IF YOU HAVE . . .
- Rotator cuff injury
- Shoulder instability

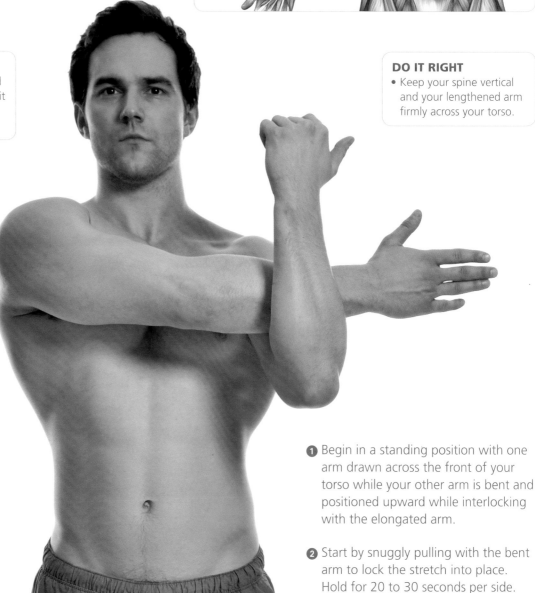

❶ Begin in a standing position with one arm drawn across the front of your torso while your other arm is bent and positioned upward while interlocking with the elongated arm.

❷ Start by snuggly pulling with the bent arm to lock the stretch into place. Hold for 20 to 30 seconds per side.

LATERAL STRETCH

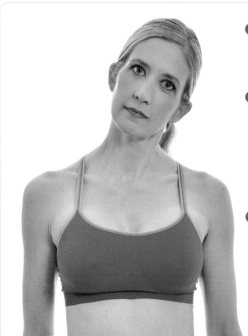

1. Sit or stand, keeping your neck, shoulders and torso straight.

2. Tilt your head so that your right ear moves toward your right shoulder until you feel a distinct stretch in the left side of your neck.

3. Hold for 10 seconds, and repeat three times in each direction.

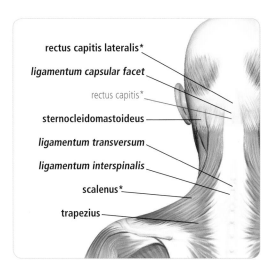

rectus capitis lateralis*
ligamentum capsular facet
rectus capitis*
sternocleidomastoideus
ligamentum transversum
ligamentum interspinalis
scalenus*
trapezius

ANNOTATION KEY

Black text indicates target muscles
Gray text indicates other working muscles
Italics indicates ligaments
* indicates deep muscles

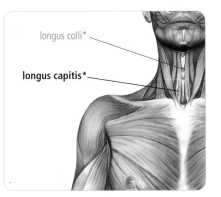

longus colli*
longus capitis*

BEST FOR

- scalenus
- sternocleidomastoideus
- trapezius
- longus capitis
- rectus capitis lateralis
- ligamentum transversum
- ligamentum interspinalis
- ligamentum capsular facet

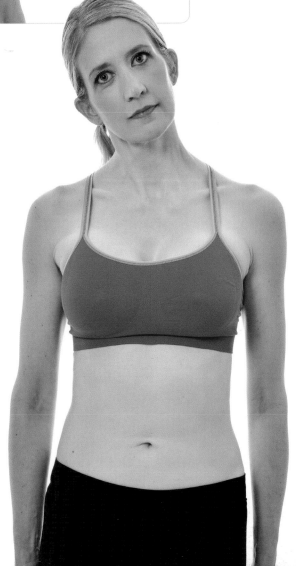

TARGETS
- Neck lateral flexors

LEVEL
- Beginner

BENEFITS
- Improves range of motion
- Relieves neck pain

NOT ADVISABLE IF YOU HAVE . . .
- Numbness running down your arm or into your hand

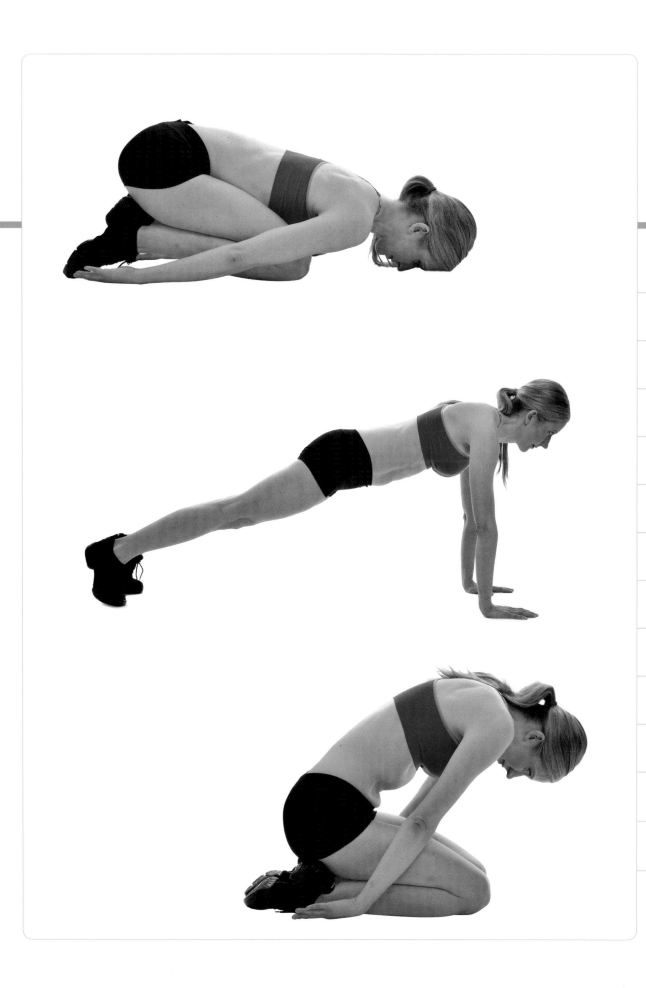

PUT IT ALL TOGETHER:
LONGEVITY WORKOUTS

Once you have gone through the seven longevity modalities illustrated in this

book and practiced executing the exercises properly, your next step is to put

these moves together. The following sequences are just samples of the many

ways that you can combine these exercises to create targeted workouts. They

provide flexible frameworks that you can adapt to accommodate your specific

fitness level or area of concern—if you want to avoid a certain exercise in

any one of them, simply substitute another that has a similar benefit. Try the

workouts featured here, and then flip through the exercises and create your

own workouts to suit your individual goals.

NEWBIE WORKOUT

This series of exercises is suitable for all levels, especially those in their later years who are new to training.

1 Child's Pose

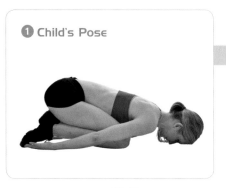

pages 80–81

2 Plank Pose

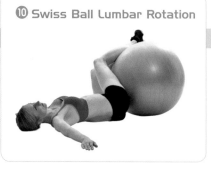

page 88

3 Swiss Ball Dumbbell Pullover

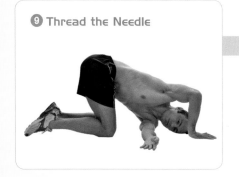

pages 32–33

4 Seated Alternating Dumbbell Press

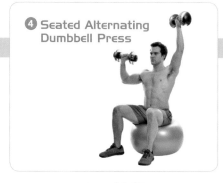

pages 34–35

5 Swiss Ball Squat with Dumbbell Curl

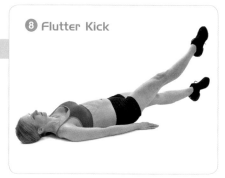

pages 26–27

6 High Knees

pages 98–99

7 Balance Walk

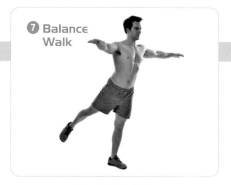

pages 124–125

8 Flutter Kick

pages 112–113

9 Thread the Needle

pages 76–77

10 Swiss Ball Lumbar Rotation

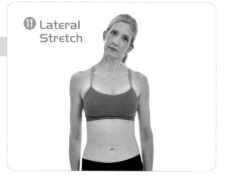

pages 62–63

11 Lateral Stretch

page 147

POSTURAL WORKOUT

This group of exercises strengthens the muscles that support your spine, which helps improve posture.

① Kneeling to Semi-Kneeling Progression

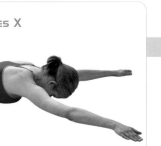

pages 46–47

② Swiss Ball Lumbar Rotation

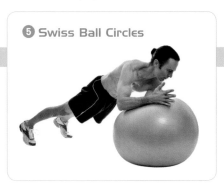

pages 62–63

③ Pelvic Side Raise

pages 48–49

④ Pilates X

pages 56–57

⑤ Swiss Ball Circles

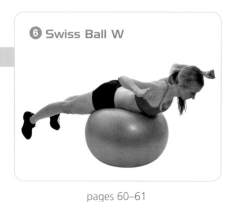

pages 58–59

⑥ Swiss Ball W

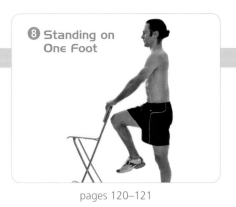

pages 60–61

⑦ Sitting Balance

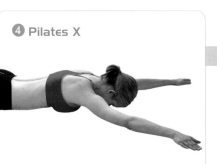

page 131

⑧ Standing on One Foot

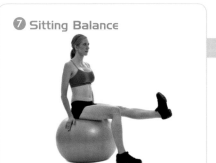

pages 120–121

⑨ Walking Heel-to-Toe

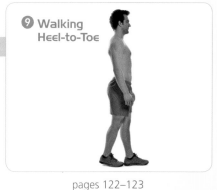

pages 122–123

⑩ Trunk Curl

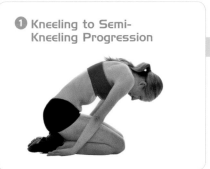

pages 50–51

⑪ Reverse Trunk Curl

pages 52–53

⑫ Flutter Kick

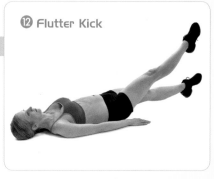

pages 112–113

STRENGTH WORKOUT

This workout, with its emphasis on improved power and explosive movement, will strengthen your entire body.

1 Inchworm

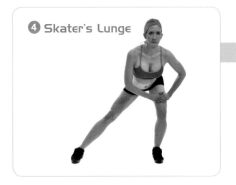

pages 100–101

2 Diver's Push-Up

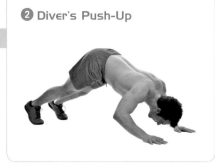

pages 104–105

3 Step-Up

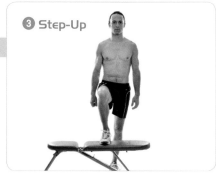

pages 106–107

4 Skater's Lunge

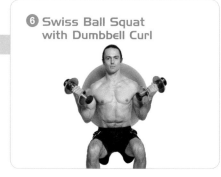

pages 108–109

5 Lateral Stepover

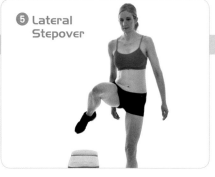

pages 110–111

6 Swiss Ball Squat with Dumbbell Curl

pages 26–27

7 Swiss Ball Incline Dumbbell Press

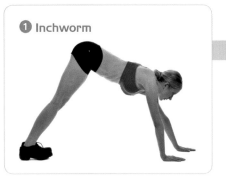

pages 30–31

8 Swiss Ball One-Arm Row

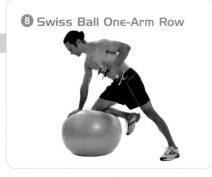

pages 126–127

9 One-Arm Swiss Ball Triceps Kickback

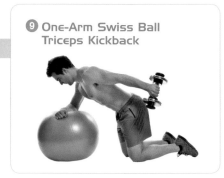

pages 36–37

10 Swiss Ball Hamstring Flexibility

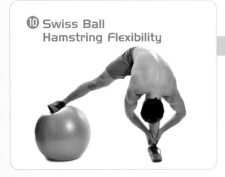

page 130

11 Swiss Ball Plank with Leg Raise

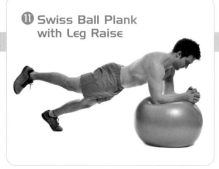

pages 132–133

12 Butterfly Stretch

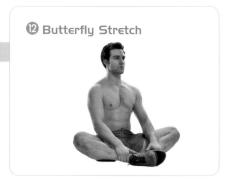

page 137

MOVE-EASY WORKOUT

Regularly performing this groups of exercises will enhance ongoing and sustained movement.

① Lunge with Dumbbell Upright Row

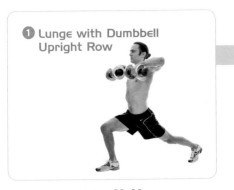

pages 28–29

② Swiss Ball Flye

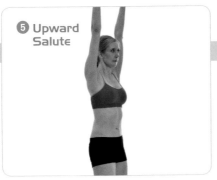

pages 40–41

③ Downward-Facing Dog

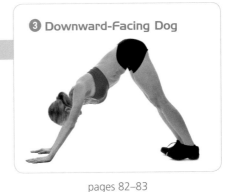

pages 82–83

④ Tree Pose

pages

page 87

⑤ Upward Salute

page 86

⑥ Chair Pose

pages 94–95

⑦ Swiss Ball Circles

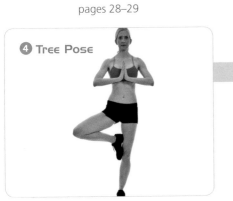

pages 58–59

⑧ Diver's Push-Up

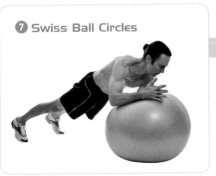

pages 104–105

⑨ High Knees

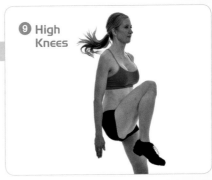

pages 98–99

⑩ Skater's Lunge

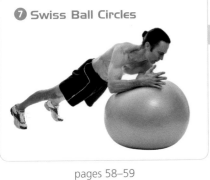

pages 108–109

⑪ Butt Kick

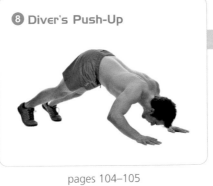

pages 102–103

⑫ Flutter Kick

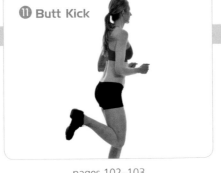

pages 112–113

TOTAL-BODY WORKOUT

This series of exercises provides a complete workout in one sitting.

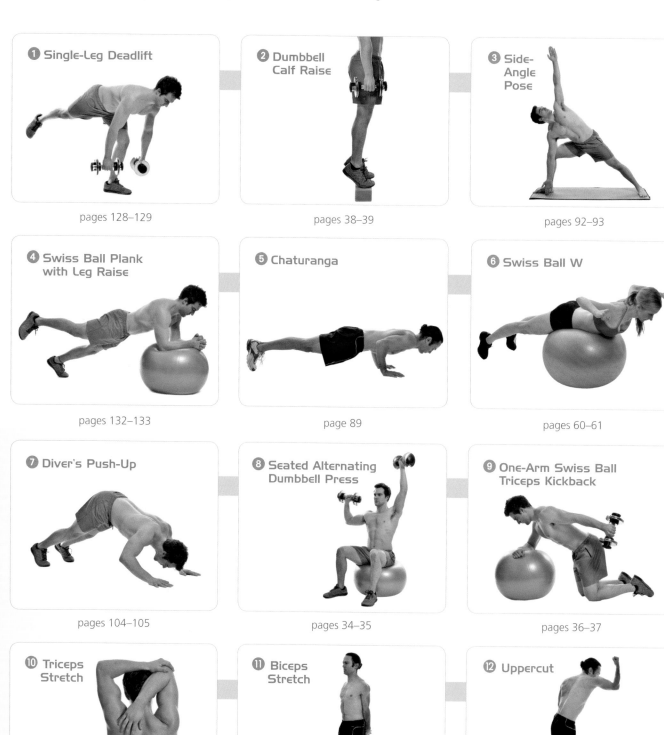

1 Single-Leg Deadlift

pages 128–129

2 Dumbbell Calf Raise

pages 38–39

3 Side-Angle Pose

pages 92–93

4 Swiss Ball Plank with Leg Raise

pages 132–133

5 Chaturanga

page 89

6 Swiss Ball W

pages 60–61

7 Diver's Push-Up

pages 104–105

8 Seated Alternating Dumbbell Press

pages 34–35

9 One-Arm Swiss Ball Triceps Kickback

pages 36–37

10 Triceps Stretch

page 142

11 Biceps Stretch

pages 143

12 Uppercut

pages 116–117

RANGE-OF-MOTION WORKOUT

Perform this workout to improve flexibility, reach and overall performance.

① Squat Test

pages 70–71

② Step-Up

pages 106–107

③ Couch Stretch

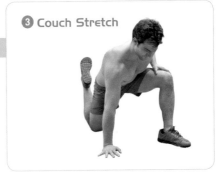

pages 66–67

④ Anterior Hip Mobilization

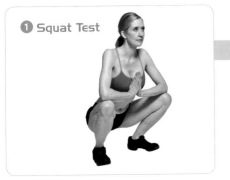

pages 72–73

⑤ External Rotation Shoulder Extension

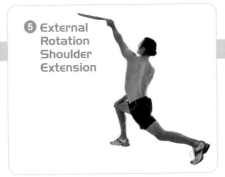

page 75

⑥ Posterior Hip Mobilization

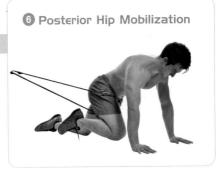

pages 68–69

⑦ Wall-Assisted Chest Stretch

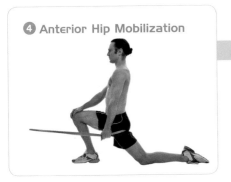

pages 144–145

⑧ Shoulder Stretch

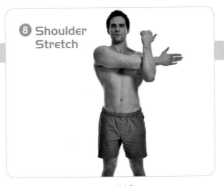

page 146

⑨ Power Punch

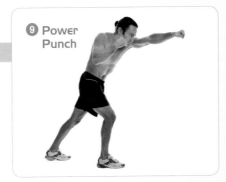

pages 114–115

⑩ Uppercut

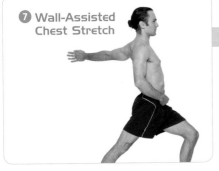

pages 116–117

⑪ Swiss Ball Rear Lateral Raise

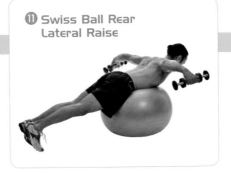

pages 42–43

⑫ Upward-Facing Dog

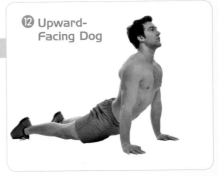

pages 90–91

CONDITIONING WORKOUT

For setting the clock back and achieving your best performance levels, try this group of exercises.

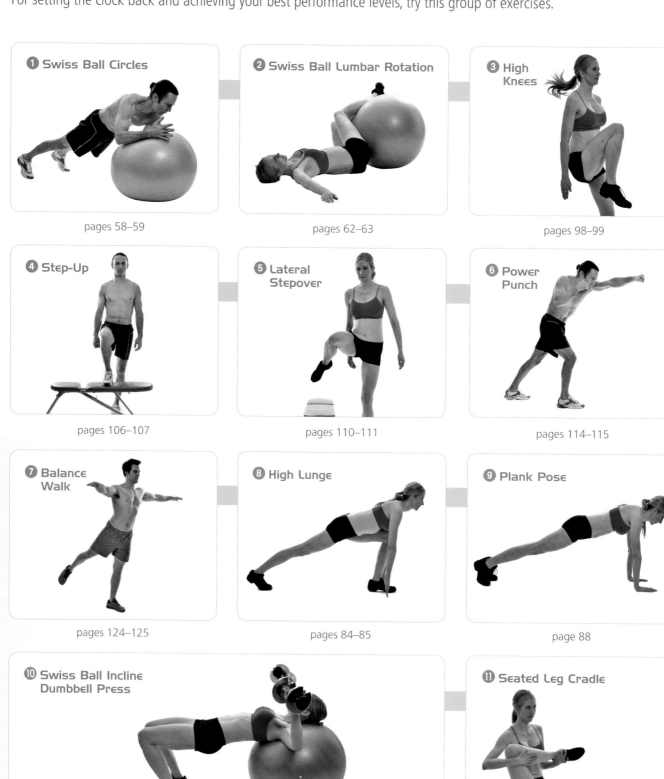

1 Swiss Ball Circles

pages 58–59

2 Swiss Ball Lumbar Rotation

pages 62–63

3 High Knees

pages 98–99

4 Step-Up

pages 106–107

5 Lateral Stepover

pages 110–111

6 Power Punch

pages 114–115

7 Balance Walk

pages 124–125

8 High Lunge

pages 84–85

9 Plank Pose

page 88

10 Swiss Ball Incline Dumbbell Press

pages 30–31

11 Seated Leg Cradle

page 136

THE NOAH'S ARK WORKOUT

This group is for those who want a sampling from the full longevity menu with a taste of everything.

❶ Lunge with Dumbbell Upright Row

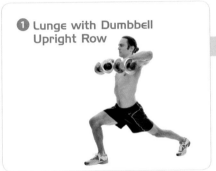

pages 28–29

❷ Swiss Ball Flye

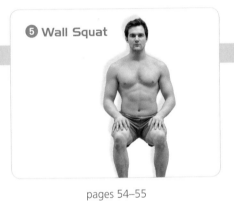

pages 40–41

❸ Tree Pose

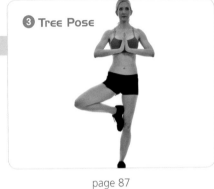

page 87

❹ Side-Angle Pose

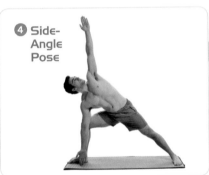

pages 92–93

❺ Wall Squat

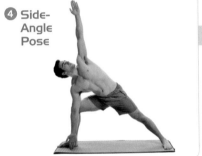

pages 54–55

❻ Ankle Dorsiflexion

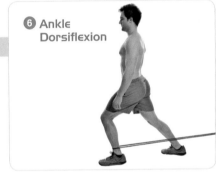

page 74

❼ Swiss Ball One-Arm Row

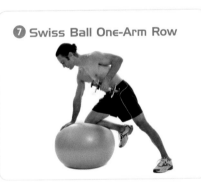

pages 126–127

❽ Skater's Lunge

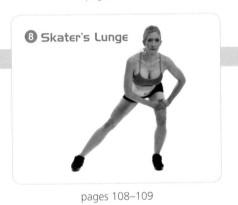

pages 108–109

❾ Flutter Kick

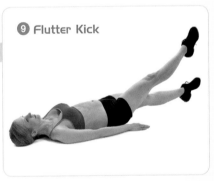

pages 112–113

❿ Side-Lying Knee Bend

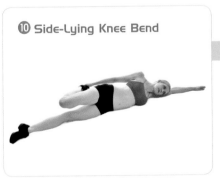

page 140

⓫ Hip and Lower-Back Stretch

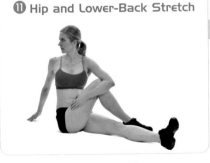

pages 138–139

⓬ Kneeling Lat Stretch

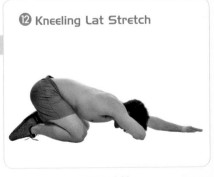

page 141

GLOSSARY

GENERAL TERMS

abduction: Movement away from the body.

adduction: Movement toward the body.

anterior: Located in the front.

cardiovascular exercise: Any exercise that increases the heart rate, making oxygen and nutrient-rich blood available to working muscles.

core: Refers to the deep muscle layers that lie close to the spine and provide structural support for the entire body. The core is divided into two groups: the major and the minor. The major muscles reside on the trunk and include the belly area and the middle and lower back. This area encompasses the pelvic floor muscles (levator ani, pubococcygeus, iliococcygeus, puborectalis and coccygeus), the abdominals (rectus abdominis, transversus abdominis, obliquus externus and obliquus internus), the spinal extensors (multifidus spinae, erector spinae, splenius, longissimus thoracis and semispinalis) and the diaphragm. The minor core muscles include the latissimus dorsi, gluteus maximus and trapezius. Minor core muscles assist the major muscles when the body engages in activities or movements that require added stability.

curl: An exercise movement, usually targeting the biceps brachii, that calls for a weight to be moved through an arc, in a "curling" motion.

deadlift: An exercise movement that calls for lifting a weight, such as a dumbbell, off the floor from a stabilized bent-over position.

dumbbell: A basic piece of equipment that consists of a short bar on which plates are secured. A person can use a dumbbell in one or both hands during an exercise. Most gyms offer dumbbells with the weight plates welded on and poundage indicated on the plates, but many dumbbells intended for home use come with removable plates that allow you to adjust the weight.

extension: The act of straightening.

extensor muscle: A muscle serving to extend a body part away from the body.

flexion: The bending of a joint.

flexor muscle: A muscle that decreases the angle between two bones, as when bending the arm at the elbow or raising the thigh toward the stomach.

flye: An exercise movement in which the hand and arm move through an arc while the elbow is kept at a constant angle. Flyes work the muscles of the upper body.

hamstrings: The three muscles of the posterior thigh (the semitendinosus, semimembranosus and biceps femoris) that work to flex the knee and extend the hip.

hand weight: Any of a range of free weights that are often used in weight training and toning. Small hand weights are usually cast iron formed in the shape of a dumbbell, sometimes coated with rubber or neoprene for comfort.

iliotibial band (ITB): A thick band of fibrous tissue that runs down the outside of the leg, beginning at the hip and extending to the outer side of the tibia just below the knee joint. The band functions in concert with several of the thigh muscles to provide stability to the outside of the knee joint.

lateral: Located on, or extending toward, the outside.

medial: Located on, or extending toward, the middle.

posterior: Located behind.

press: An exercise movement that calls for moving a weight or other resistance away from the body.

quadriceps: A large muscle group (full name: quadriceps femoris) that includes the four prevailing muscles on the front of the thigh: the rectus femoris, vastus intermedius, vastus lateralis and vastus medialis. It is the great extensor muscle of the knee, forming a large fleshy mass that covers the front and sides of the femur muscle.

range of motion: The distance and direction a joint can move between the flexed and the extended positions.

resistance band: Any rubber tubing or flat band device that provides a resistive force used for strength training. Also called a "fitness band," "Thera-Band," "Dyna-Band," "stretching band," and "exercise band."

rotator muscle: One of a group of muscles that assist the rotation of a joint, such as the hip or the shoulder.

squat: An exercise movement that calls for moving the hips back and bending the knees and hips to lower the torso and an accompanying weight, and then returning to the upright position. A squat primarily targets the muscles of the thighs, hips, buttocks and hamstrings.

Swiss ball: A flexile, inflatable PVC ball measuring approximately 12 to 30 incehs (30–76 cm) in circumference that is used for weight training, physical therapy, balance training and many other exercise regimens. It is also called a "balance ball," "fitness ball," "stability ball," "exercise ball," "gym ball," "physioball," "body ball," "therapy ball" and many other names.

warm-up: Any form of light exercise of short duration that prepares the body for more intense exercises.

weight: Refers to the plates or weight stacks, or the actual poundage listed on the bar or dumbbell.

LATIN TERMS
The following glossary explains the Latin scientific terminology used to describe the muscles of the human body. Certain words are derived from Greek, which is indicated in each instance.

CHEST

coracobrachialis: Greek *korakoeidés*, "ravenlike," and *brachium*, "arm"

pectoralis (major and minor): *pectus*, "breast"

ABDOMEN

obliquus (externus and internus): *obliquus*, "slanting"

rectus abdominis: *rego*, "straight, upright," and *abdomen*, "belly"

serratus anterior: *serra*, "saw," and *ante*, "before"

transversus abdominis: *transversus*, "athwart," and *abdomen*, "belly"

NECK

scalenus: Greek *skalénós*, "unequal"

semispinalis: *semi*, "half," and *spinae*, "spine"

splenius: Greek *splénion*, "plaster, patch"

sternocleidomastoideus: Greek *stérnon*, "chest," Greek *kleís*, "key" and Greek *mastoeidés*, "breastlike"

BACK

erector spinae: *erectus*, "straight," and *spina*, "thorn"

latissimus dorsi: *latus*, "wide," and *dorsum*, "back"

multifidus spinae: *multifid*, "to cut into divisions," and *spinae*, "spine"

quadratus lumborum: *quadratus*, "square, rectangular," and *lumbus*, "loin"

rhomboideus: Greek *rhembesthai*, "to spin"

trapezius: Greek *trapezion*, "small table"

SHOULDERS

deltoideus (anterior, medialis and posterior): Greek *deltoeidés*, "delta-shaped"

infraspinatus: *infra*, "under," and *spina*, "thorn"

levator scapulae: *levare*, "to raise," and *scapulae*, "shoulder [blades]"

subscapularis: *sub*, "below," and *scapulae*, "shoulder [blades]"

supraspinatus: *supra*, "above," and *spina*, "thorn"

teres (major and minor): *teres*, "rounded"

UPPER ARM

biceps brachii: *biceps*, "two-headed," and *brachium*, "arm"

brachialis: *brachium*, "arm"

triceps brachii: *triceps*, "three-headed" and *brachium*, "arm"

LOWER ARM

anconeus: Greek *anconad*, "elbow"

brachioradialis: *brachium*, "arm," and *radius*, "spoke"

extensor carpi radialis: *extendere*, "to extend," Greek *karpós*, "wrist" and *radius*, "spoke"

extensor digitorum: *extendere*, "to extend," and *digitus*, "finger, toe"

flexor carpi pollicis longus: *flectere*, "to bend," Greek *karpós*, "wrist," *pollicis*, "thumb" and *longus*, "long"

flexor carpi radialis: *flectere*, "to bend," Greek *karpós*, "wrist" and *radius*, "spoke"

flexor carpi ulnaris: *flectere*, "to bend," Greek *karpós*, "wrist" and *ulnaris*, "forearm"

flexor digitorum: *flectere*, "to bend," and *digitus*, "finger, toe"

palmaris longus: *palmaris*, "palm," and *longus*, "long"

pronator teres: *pronate*, "to rotate," and *teres*, "rounded"

HIPS

gemellus (inferior and superior): *geminus*, "twin"

gluteus maximus: Greek *gloutós*, "rump," and *maximus*, "largest"

gluteus medius: Greek *gloutós*, "rump" and *medialis*, "middle"

gluteus minimus: Greek *gloutós*, "rump" and *minimus*, "smallest"

iliopsoas: *ilium*, "groin," and Greek *psoa*, "groin muscle"

obturator externus: *obturare*, "to block" and *externus*, "outward"

obturator internus: *obturare*, "to block," and *internus*, "within"

pectineus: *pectin*, "comb"

piriformis: *pirum*, "pear," and *forma*, "shape"

quadratus femoris: *quadratus*, "square, rectangular," and *femur*, "thigh"

UPPER LEG

adductor longus: *adducere*, "to contract," and *longus*, "long"

adductor magnus: *adducere*, "to contract," and *magnus*, "major"

biceps femoris: *biceps*, "two-headed," and *femur*, "thigh"

gracilis: *gracilis*, "slim, slender"

rectus femoris: *rego*, "straight, upright," and *femur*, "thigh"

sartorius: *sarcio*, "to patch" or "to repair"

semimembranosus: *semi*, "half," and *membrum*, "limb"

semitendinosus: *semi*, "half," and *tendo*, "tendon"

tensor fasciae latae: *tenere*, "to stretch," *fasciae*, "band," and *latae*, "laid down"

vastus intermedius: *vastus*, "immense, huge," and *intermedius*, "between"

vastus lateralis: *vastus*, "immense, huge," and *lateralis*, "side"

vastus medialis: *vastus*, "immense, huge," and *medialis*, "middle"

LOWER LEG

adductor digiti minimi: *adducere*, "to contract," *digitus*, "finger, toe" and *minimum* "smallest"

adductor hallucis: *adducere*, "to contract," and *hallex*, "big toe"

extensor digitorum longus: *extendere*, "to extend," *digitus*, "finger, toe" and *longus*, "long"

extensor hallucis longus: *extendere*, "to extend," *hallex*, "big toe," and *longus*, "long"

flexor digitorum longus: *flectere*, "to bend," *digitus*, "finger, toe" and *longus*, "long"

flexor hallucis longus: *flectere*, "to bend," and *hallex*, "big toe" and *longus*, "long"

gastrocnemius: Greek *gastroknémia*, "calf [of the leg]"

peroneus: *peronei*, "of the fibula"

plantaris: *planta*, "the sole"

soleus: *solea*, "sandal"

tibialis (anterior and posterior): *tibia*, "reed pipe"

CREDITS & ACKNOWLEDGMENTS

All photographs by Jonathan Conklin/Jonathan Conklin Photography, Inc. (jonathanconklin.net), except the following pages: 8 Monkey Business Images/Shutterstock.com; 10 bikeriderlondon/Shutterstock.com; 12 Monkey Business Images/Shutterstock.com; 13 T-Design/Shutterstock.com; 14 Robert Kneschke/Shutterstock.com; 15 (left) Lisovskaya Natalia/Shutterstock.com; 15 (right) Evgeny Karandaev/Shutterstock.com;16 Elena Ray/Shutterstock.com; 17 Gelpi JM/Shutterstock.com; 18 racorn/Shutterstock.com; 19 Monkey Business Images/Shutterstock.com; 20 Monkey Business Images/Shutterstock.com; 21 (box left) picamaniac/Shutterstock.com; 32 (box) Philip Date/Shutterstock.com; 36 (box) Philip Date/Shutterstock.com; 61 (box) Philip Date/Shutterstock.com; 129 (box) Philip Date/Shutterstock.com

Models: BJ Gruber, David MacManamon, Lou Matthews and Elaine Altholz

All large anatomical illustrations by Hector Aiza/3D Labz Animation India (www.3dlabz.com), with small insets by Linda Bucklin/Shutterstock.com.

Acknowledgments

The author and publisher also offer thanks to those closely involved in the creation of this book: Moseley Road president Sean Moore; project editor and designer Lisa Purcell; consultant Katerina Spilio; production designer Adam Moore; and photographer Jonathan Conklin.

About the Author

Before his career as author and personal trainer, Hollis Lance Liebman had been a fitness magazine editor, national bodybuilding champion and published physique photographer, and he has also served as a bodybuilding and fitness competition judge. Currently a Los Angeles resident, Hollis has worked with some of Hollywood's elite, earning himself rave reviews.

Visit www.holliswashere.com to keep up with all of his latest fitness tips and complete training programs.